Atlas and Synopsis
of
Contact and Occupational Dermatology

Atlas and Synopsis
of
Contact and Occupational
Dermatology

Sanjay Ghosh MD
Medical Director
Institute of Allergic and Immunologic
Skin Diseases
Kolkata
India

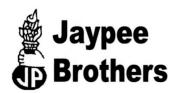

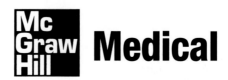

© 2009, Jaypee Brothers Medical Publishers

First published in India in 2009 by

Jaypee Brothers Medical Publishers (P) Ltd

Corporate Office
4838/24 Ansari Road, Daryaganj, **New Delhi** - 110002, India, +91-11-43574357

Registered Office
B-3 EMCA House, 23/23B Ansari Road, Daryaganj, **New Delhi** 110 002, India
Phones: +91-11-23272143, +91-11-23272703, +91-11-23282021,
+91-11-23245672, Rel: +91-11-32558559 Fax: +91-11-23276490, +91-11-23245683
e-mail: jaypee@jaypeebrothers.com, Website: www.jaypeebrothers.com

First published in USA by The McGraw-Hill Companies, 2 Penn Plaza, New York, NY 10121. Exclusively
worldwide distributor except South Asia (India, Nepal, Sri Lanka, Bhutan, Pakistan, Bangladesh, Malaysia).

ISBN-13: 978-0-07-163230-0
ISBN-10: 0-07-163230-1

To
My daughter
Shinjini

Foreword

Globally, contact and occupational dermatoses are common skin disorders. There are a large number of exogenous hazardous factors which may cause a great variety of skin manifestations from eczema to depigmentation and skin cancer. The spectrum of hazardous factors is constantly changing with introduction of, for example, new sensitizing chemicals. There are also geographical differences in the presence and exposure to hazardous factors which make this book with an Asian perspective a valuable resource to instruct and help all who read it and hopefully also stimulate many to take a greater interest in this fascinating area.

Magnus Bruze
Professor
Department of Occupational and
Environmental Dermatology
University Hospital
Malmö
Sweden

Preface

During my last twenty three years 'live-together' (I dare to say 'marriage' because of my wife!) with the subject dermatology I felt many a time that contact and occupational dermatology remains a low-profile subset of dermatology in spite of the fact that each and every dermatologist has to deal with quite a good number of these type of patients in their daily practice. This applies to any dermatologist from any set up; urban or rural, tertiary or secondary health care hospitals. Moreover, in recent years, due to rapid urbanisation and fast life pattern changes, the horizon of the subject has been widened considerably. Conception regarding the diseases is becoming more distinct; newer disease entities on this topic have been described. The suffering and work-day loss due to contact and occupational dermatoses create a tremendous impact on the health system of any nation. However, the shining glamour and easy-money of the subjects like dermatosurgery and cosmetology have recently attracted many young dermatologists towards them whereas less sounding contact and occupational dermatology, which had gained its importance as super-speciality much earlier compared with these newer subjects, remains a bit under-practised and neglected especially in our country.

In the postgraduate syllabus this subject is often not stressed upon that much. Practical knowledge about patch test, interpretation of its result sometimes remain unknown to a postgraduate student passing final examination in dermatology! Students often feel disinterested about the subject as they think contact and occupational dermatology means only some long chemical names! The books on the subject, especially in perspective of our country, are really sparse.

The above thinking process has led me to write a book on this subject. But as dermatology is more a visual subject and could be more interesting if written in atlas form I decided to provide the information in 'Atlas and Synopsis' pattern. However, this book is never a substitute of bigger textbooks and treatises on this subject. Above all this book has not been written by assuming the specialists working in this field as the main readers. Rather the dermatologists, who see all type of skin cases in daily practice but sometimes face difficulty to deal cases of contact or occupational dermatoses and the postgraduate students are the probable target readers of this book. The details of the subject especially histopathology and immunology of contact dermatitis have been purposefully omitted which can be best consulted in any standard book on this subject. Footwear dermatitis, airborne contact dermatitis, cosmetic and medicament dermatitis have been discussed in detail as they are quite common in Indian scenario. A chapter on chemical leukoderma has been included as this disease is induced primarily by contact with the offending chemicals although the etiomechanism is different from contact dermatitis. Moreover this ailment represents an important subset of the occupational dermatology.

In writing this book I am indebted to the whole medical team of our Institute of Allergic and Immunological Skin Diseases, who are constantly engaged in the specialized job of dealing the cases of contact and occupational dermatology. They are Dr Manas Sen, Dr Dinesh Hawelia, Dr Susmit Haldar, Dr Sukti Mukhopadhyaya, Dr Nilendu Sarma, Dr Sanjib Chowdhury and Dr Sudip Kr Ghosh. I must acknowledge Mr. Subhrajyoti Bose for organizing all the technical matters related to this book. Last but not the least I feel grateful to my wife Mrs Shrabani Ghosh and my daughter Ms Shinjini Ghosh for constantly bearing me and providing constant enthusiasm for this obsessive effort.

Sanjay Ghosh

Dial : +91 033 2442 8011, 9831085082

E-mail: drsanjayg@dataone.in

Contents

1 Classification of Contact Dermatitis

Contact dermatitis denotes superficial inflammation of the skin induced by exogenous chemicals interacting on the skin.

Like other forms of dermatitis contact dermatitis can represent any of the three phases: acute, subacute or chronic. One form may merge into another form by evolution.

> Phases of contact dermatitis:
> - Acute
> - Subacute
> - Chronic

On the basis of etiopathogenesis contact dermatitis can be of two types: irritant contact dermatitis and allergic contact dermatitis.

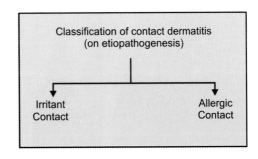

Classification of contact dermatitis
(on etiopathogenesis)

Irritant Contact

Allergic Contact

PHASES OF CONTACT DERMATITIS

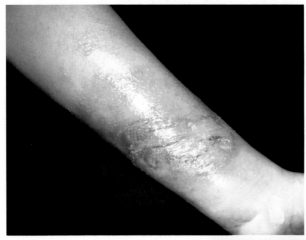

<u>FIGURE 1.1</u>
Acute phase : oozing, vesiculation

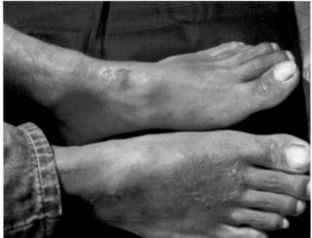

<u>FIGURE 1.2</u>
Subacute phase: less oozing, less
vesiculation, scaling, mild lichenification

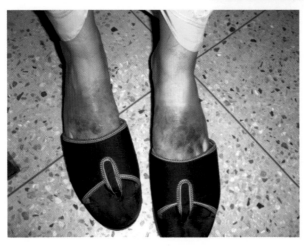

<u>FIGURE 1.3</u>
Chronic phase: marked lichenification,
hyperkeratosis, no vesiculation, no oozing

Irritant contact dermatitis (80%) is much common than allergic contact dermatitis (20%).

Although the two types of contact dermatitis differ conceptually their cellular and cytokines profiles bear very close resemblance. Their basic difference is in the antigen specificity; allergic contact dermatitis possesses this specificity whereas irritant contact dermatitis does not possess this.

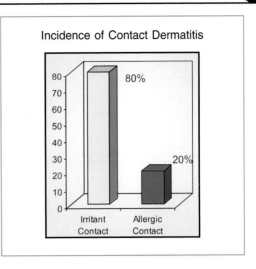

Incidence of Contact Dermatitis

Comparison between Irritant and Allergic Contact Dermatitis		
	Irritant contact dermatitis	*Allergic contact dermatitis*
1. Antigen-specificity	Non-specific	Specific
2. Sensitization	Not required	Required
3. Genetic predisposition	Not present	Present
4. Pruritus	Not marked (early)	Marked
5. Pain/Burning	Pronounced (early)	Less pronounced
6. Vesicles	Not common	Common
7. Pustules	Common	Not common

2 Irritant Contact Dermatitis

Irritant contact dermatitis can be classified into two stages: Acute irritant contact dermatitis and cumulative irritant contact dermatitis.

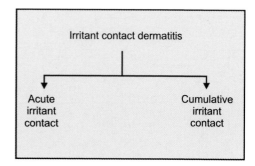

	Acute irritant	Cumulative irritant
Acute Irritant Contact Versus Cumulative Irritant Contact Dermatitis		
1. Number of chemical insult	Usually single	Multiple
2. Nature of chemical	Strong irritants, (Concentrated alkali or acid, strong solvent, strong oxidising or reducing agents, etc.)	Weak irritant (water, detergent, weak, solvents, oils or greases)
3. Nature of damage	Toxic cell damage	Cumulative wear and tear
4. Evolution	Erythema → vesiculation (sometime not present) → exudation → crusting → scaling → residual erythema → post-inflammatory hyperpigmentation	Chronic throughout
5. Demarcation	Sharp	Diffuse

CRITERIA FOR DIAGNOSIS OF IRRITANT CONTACT DERMATITIS

A. Subjective Criteria

Major

1. Symptoms start instantly

2. Pain, burning, stinging or discomfort predominate rather than pruritus

Minor

1. Onset of the dermatitis within 2 weeks of exposure

2. Many people in the environment similarly affected

B. Objective Criteria

Major

1. Macular erythema, hyperkeratosis or fissuring more common than vesicular changes
2. Glazed, scalded or parched look
3. The healing process starts without plateau upon withdrawal of the offending agent
4. Patch test shows negative result

Minor

1. Sharply demarcated lesion
2. Evidence of gravitational influence, e.g. dripping effect
3. Localised lesion (not much spreading)
4. Vesicles closely juxtaposed to patches of erythema, erosions, bullae, etc

(Rietshel R, 1990)

ACUTE IRRITANT CONTACT DERMATITIS

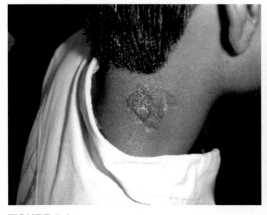

FIGURE 2.1

Acute irritant contact dermatitis on neck after application of a pain-relieving strong balm (counter-irritant)

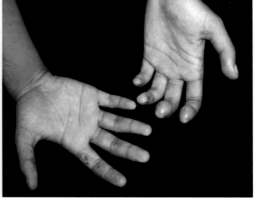

FIGURE 2.2

Acute irritant dermititis on both hands of a student after contacting strong alkali during his chemistry practical procedure in school

ACUTE LRRITANT CONTACT DERMATITIS: DIFFERENT PHASES

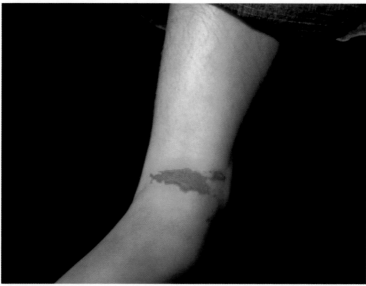

FIGURE 2.3

Early phase of acute irritant dermatitis after exposure to strong acid spilled over leg during work in a factory (Note: the sharp demarcation of the lesion)

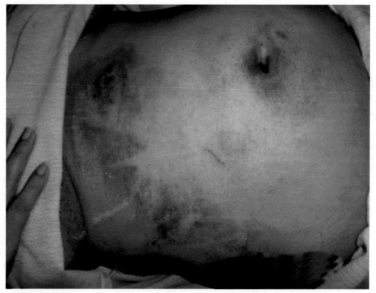

FIGURE 2.4

Late phase of acute irritant contact dermatitis in a lady who was using undiluted, strong antiseptic (savlon) to wash her abdominal wounds caused by laparoscopy for cholecystectomy

CUMULATIVE IRRITANT CONTACT DERMATITIS

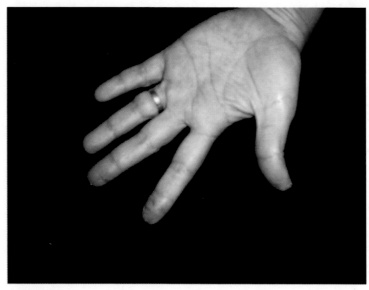

FIGURE 2.5

Cumulative irritant contact dermatitis of a housewife at her fingertips due to regular contact with detergents, spices, condiments, vegetables and plants

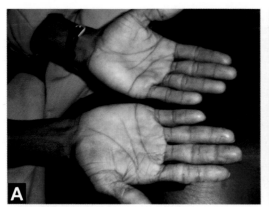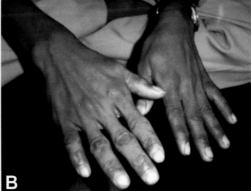

FIGURES 2.6A AND B

Cumulative irritant contact dermatitis of a person who has been working in a sweet (candy) manufacturing factory for last 20 years with regular exposure to detergents and washing soaps

3 Allergic Contact Dermatitis

Allergic contact dermatitis (ACD) represents a classic delayed hypersensitivity or a type IV immunologic reaction mediated by T lymphocytes. Immune cells rather than antibodies play major role in its pathogenesis.

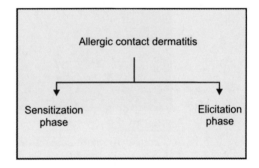

Allergic contact dermatitis to a particular agent can develop only in subjects who have been previously exposed to the substance, and have acquired a sensitization from that substance.

Allergic contact dermatitis has two phases: sensitization phase and elicitation phase.

Sensitization and Elicitation Phase of ACD	
Sensitization phase	*Elicitation phase*
1. During this phase patients acquire allergic sensitization.	1. Onset of allergy in already sensitized person
2. Latent period: Variable (upto year) Minimum : 4 days.	2. Latent period: Usually 48-72 hours

Myths and Facts Regarding Allergic Contact Dermatitis

Myths	Facts
1. Allergy develops only to new substances	1. Allergy can occur after years of contact
2. Allergy occurs immediately after contact	2. Allergy occurs almost in all cases after 1 to 2 days and sometimes appears even after a week
3. Allergy depends on the quantity of allergens (dose-dependent)	3. Allergy does not depend on the amount of allergens (not dose-dependent)
4. Allergy always occurs only at the site of contact	4. Allergy can develop in distant area (like nail polish causing ACD on eyelids). Moreover, apart from the site of contact, allergy develops at distant areas of skin by lymphatic or hematogenous dissemination of sensitizing cells
5. Negative scratch test, RAST test or prick test rules out allergic contact dermatitis	5. Only patch test is the diagnostic of allergic contact dermatitis
6. Allergic contact dermatitis is always bilateral	6. Even bilateral exposure to offending substances can lead to unilateral allergic contact dermatitis
7. ACD is not patchy	7. ACD can be patchy
8. ACD does not affect palms and soles	8. ACD can affect palms and soles
9. Using same brand of personal products allergy would not develop	9. Same personal brand can change their constituents and thus can create new allergy
10. When change of offending cosmetic substances does not cure contact dermatitis, diagnosis of contact dermatitis proves to be wrong	10. Different cosmetic substances may contain same or cross-reacting ingredients. Thus change of cosmetic does not always provide benefit
11. Expensive products are not allergenic	11. Allergy is not cost dependent
12. Age-old cosmetics (boric acid, etc.) or medicaments (mercurochrome) cannot cause allergy	12. Many older generation cosmetics or medicaments can cause allergy

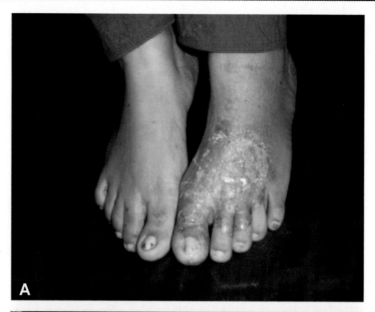

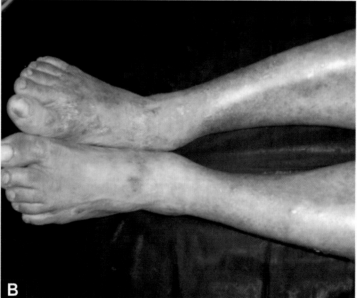

FIGURES 3.1A AND B

Allergic contact dermatitis originating from shoes affected unilaterally or predominantly one foot

THE ALLERGIC CONTACT DERMATITIS SYNDROME (ACDS)

The allergic contact dermatitis syndrome (ACDS) has three stages:

Stage 1 : Skin symptoms and signs are limited to site(s) of exposure of contact allergen(s).

Stage 2 : Regional dissemination of symptoms and signs (via lymphatic vessels), extending from the site of application of allergen(s).

Stage 3 : A. Hematogenous dissemination of symptoms and signs at a distance.

B. Systemic reactivation of allergic contact dermatitis.

> Patch test is the principal proof of diagnosis in all stages of ACDS

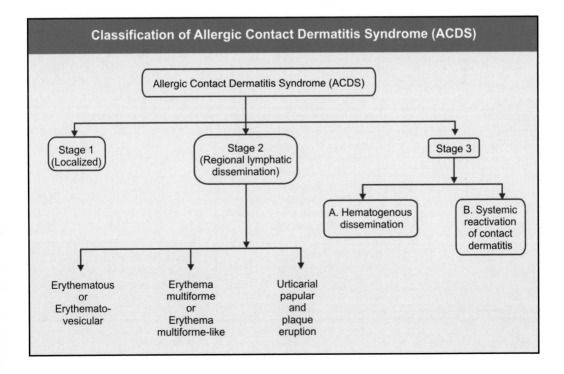

Classification of Allergic Contact Dermatitis Syndrome (ACDS)

Allergic Contact Dermatitis Syndrome (ACDS)

Stage 1 (Localized)

Stage 2 (Regional lymphatic dissemination)

Stage 3

A. Hematogenous dissemination

B. Systemic reactivation of contact dermatitis

Erythematous or Erythemato-vesicular

Erythema multiforme or Erythema multiforme-like

Urticarial papular and plaque eruption

Different Variations of Stage 1 Allergic Contact Dermatitis Syndrome (ACDS)

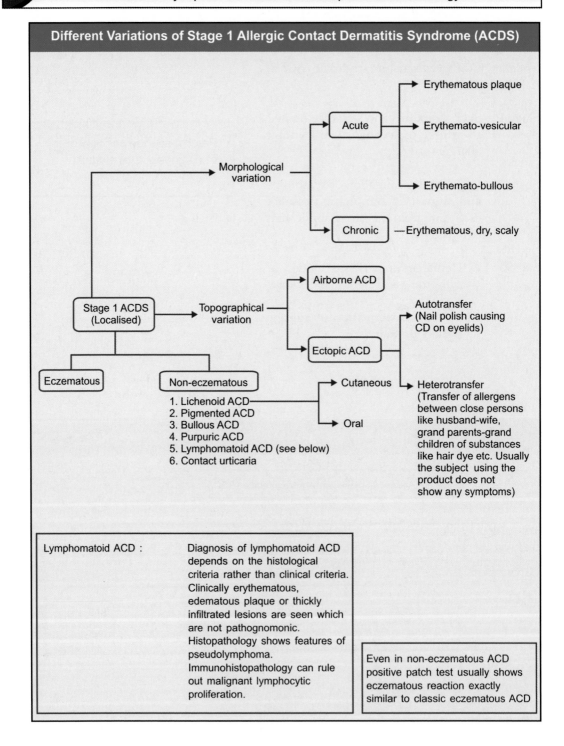

Lymphomatoid ACD :   Diagnosis of lymphomatoid ACD depends on the histological criteria rather than clinical criteria. Clinically erythematous, edematous plaque or thickly infiltrated lesions are seen which are not pathognomonic. Histopathology shows features of pseudolymphoma. Immunohistopathology can rule out malignant lymphocytic proliferation.

Even in non-eczematous ACD positive patch test usually shows eczematous reaction exactly similar to classic eczematous ACD

Stage 1 ACDS

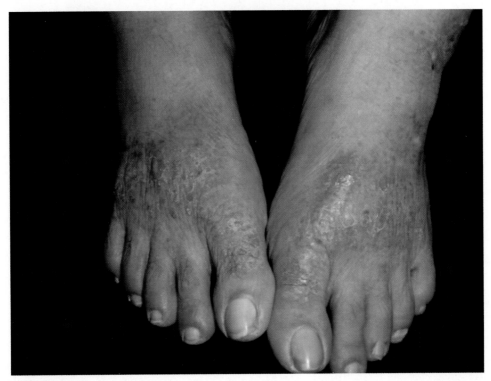

FIGURE 3.2

Allergic contact dermatitis from shoes remained localised to the site of exposure

Stage 2 ACDS

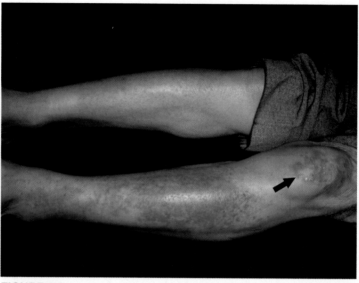

FIGURE 3.3

Primary site on legs: Secondary lymphatic dissemination to knee causing erythemato-vesicular form eruption

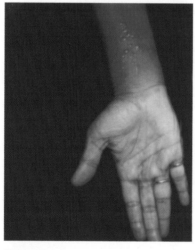

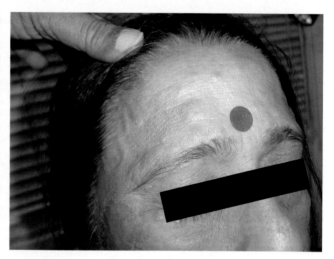

FIGURE 3.4

Secondary lymphatic dissemination to form erythema multiforme-like eruption of palm from primary site on right wrist

FIGURE 3.5

Urticarial plaques and papules on forehead from primary eczematous site of PPD allergy at the side of the face

Stage 3A ACDS

From the primary site of exposure of allergen generalized hematogenous dissemination can occur inducing secondary (or "ide") eruption. These eruptions are usually symmetrical. They present as erythematous, sometimes plaque and rarely vesicular or scaly lesions. These may erupt as 'pompholyx-type' on palmar and/or plantar surface.

> Both stage II and IIIA ACD, i.e. lymphatic and hematogenous dissemination can set in simultaneously from the primary site.

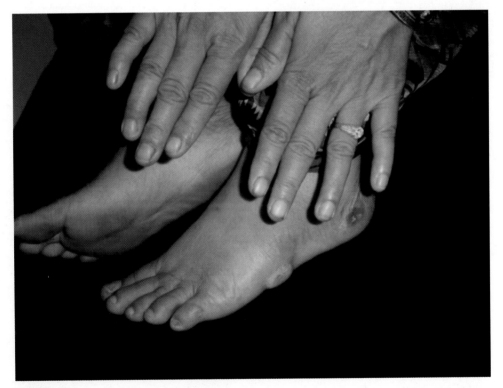

FIGURE 3.6

Allergic contact dermatitis of feet causing secondary eruption on hands. The lady had been suffering from plantar contact dermatitis for last 3 years whereas her palmar eruption had started during last 4 months only

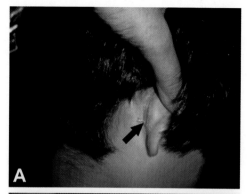

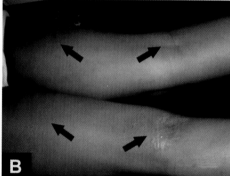

FIGURES 3.7A AND B

Primary site of involvement of post-auricular area by spectacle frame causing secondary hematogenous spread to distant flexor area of lower limbs and back of thighs

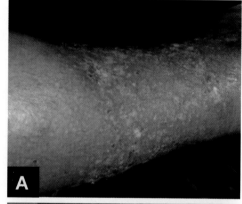

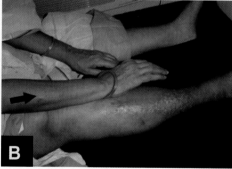

FIGURES 3.8A AND B

Primary site of involvement of lower leg (stasis dermatitis) causing hematogenous dissemination to distant area of forearms

Stage 3 B. Systemic Reactivation of Contact Dermatitis (SRCD) or Systemic Contact Dermatitis

Features

Previous episode
- Previous history of well-defined contact dermatitis weeks or even years before

Present episode
- Present history of systemic introduction of allergens or cross-reactive allergens by ingestion, inhalation or injection
- Generalised skin eruption in a symmetrical pattern.

> The only difference between Stage 3A and 3B ACDS is that presently there is no skin contact with the offending allergen in stage 3B ACDS

> The difference between stage 3B ACDS and adverse cutaneous drug reaction (ACDR) is that in ACDR the drug allergens have never been applied previously on the skin causing stage 1 ACDS

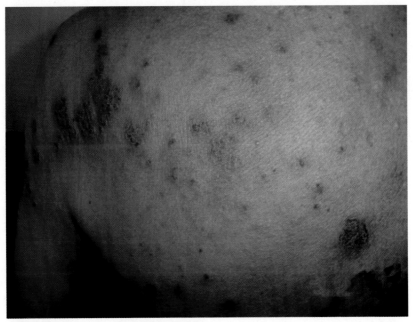

FIGURE 3.9
The patient having previous history of patch test positive-ethylenediamine allergic sensitivity developed rash of SRCD when given systemic injection of aminophylline (cross reacting with ethylenediamine)

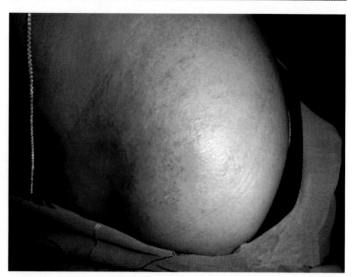

FIGURE 3.10

The patient, having previous history of allergic contact dermatitis to neem leaves on skin when touched, developed acute generalised systemic eruption when taken oral 'neem capsule' as medicine

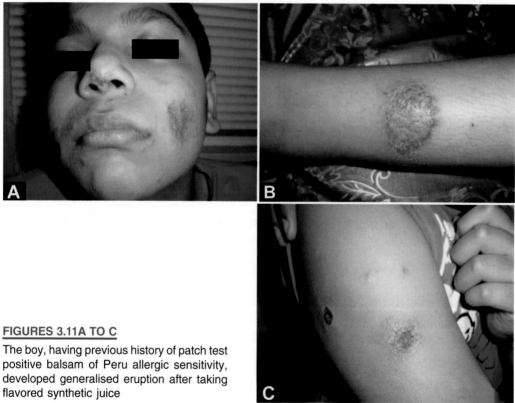

FIGURES 3.11A TO C

The boy, having previous history of patch test positive balsam of Peru allergic sensitivity, developed generalised eruption after taking flavored synthetic juice

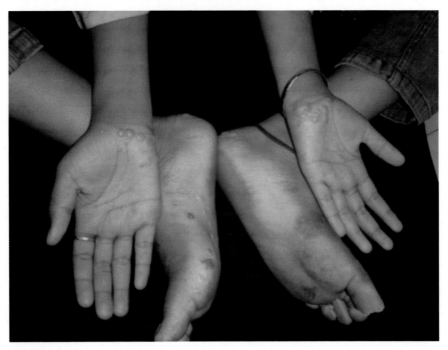

FIGURE 3.12
Recurrent palmoplantar vesicular eruption of 'pompholyx-type' of a young boy whose patch test showed positivity to nickel although he had no direct skin contact with nickel-containing agents recently. His food containing nickel (wheat flour, rice, beans, nuts, dark chocolate, etc) and nickel plates and glass used as food and drinks utensils may provoke this 'SRCD' type of eruption

Allergic patch test remains the cornerstone in the diagnosis of systemic reactivation of contact dermatitis (SRCD)

SRCD should be always kept in mind in the differential diagnosis of the following skin conditions:
1. Non-specific or 'allergic rashes'
2. Extensive eczematous eruption
3. Vesicular palmoplantar eczema or 'pompholyx'
4. 'Idiopathic' urticaria
5. Perioral eczema and cheilitis
6. Erythema multiforme
7. Vasculitis
8. Erythroderma

AIRBORNE CONTACT DERMATITIS

Airborne contact dermatitis (ABCD) implies a unique type of contact dermatitis originating from dust, sprays, pollens or volatile chemicals by airborne fumes or particles without directly handling these allergens. This form of dermatitis commonly involves face, neck, V-area of chest and eyelids. Exposed as well as non-exposed skin can be affected. Axillae and waist lines can also be the target of this disease. This form of dermatitis can sometimes be generalized.

> ABCD does not spare shadow-area like submental area contrary to phototoxic or photoallergic dermatitis

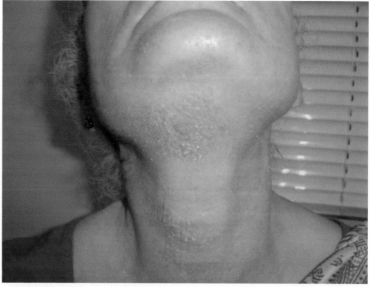

FIGURE 3.13
Submental area is also involved in airborne contact dermatitis

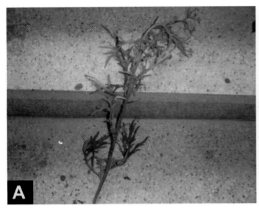
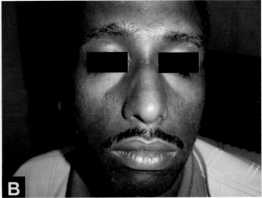

FIGURES 3.14A AND B
Airborne contact dermatitis in a patient who showed patch test positive response to parthenium

Airborne contact dermatitis in Indian patients has been attributed commonly by pollens of the plants like *Parthenium hysterophorus, Xanthium strumarium, Chrysanthemum coronarium, Helianthus annuus* (sunflower) and *Dahlia pinnata* (Nandakishore and Pasricha 1994; Pasricha and Verma 2001)

Recently cement, perfumes or deodorants, volatile paints and synthetic glues have also been described to be the contributor of ABCD especially in urban areas (Ghosh S, 2005)

Airborne contact dermatitis can be irritant airborne contact and allergic airborne contact type. They have no clinical distinction. Only patch test can distinguish between the two.

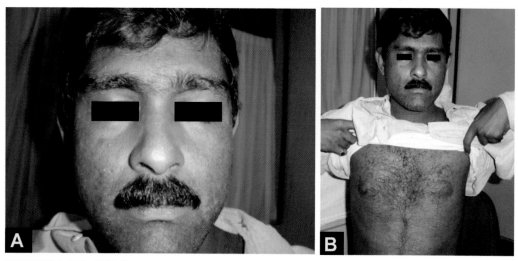

FIGURES 3.15A AND B
Airborne contact dermatitis involving face and chest originating from cement dust in a construction supervisor who does not directly handle any cement

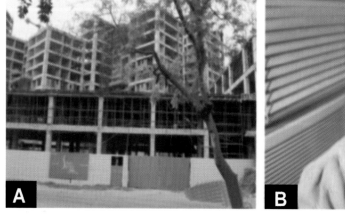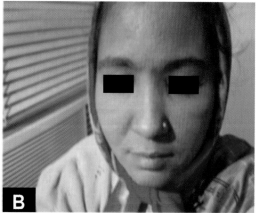

FIGURES 3.16A AND B
Airborne contact dermititis involving face of a housewife induced by cement dust whose house stands just near a vast housing projects undergoing new construction

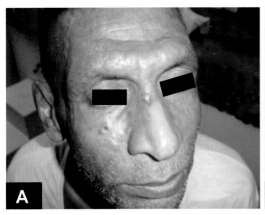 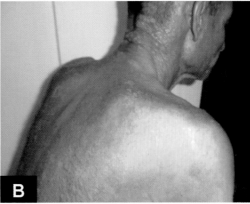

FIGURES 3.17A AND B
Airborne contact dermatitis involving face and trunk of a patient who has been working as a store-keeper in an electricity plant emitting lots of 'fly ash' though he never handled 'fly-ash' himself

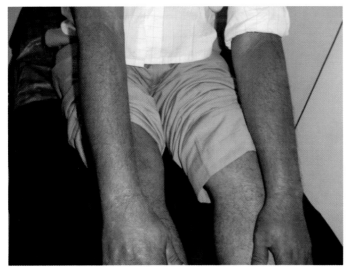

FIGURE 3.18
Airborne contact dermatitis involving forearms and legs of a quality control inspector of paint factories due to volatile paints. He frequently visits the paint factories but never handles the paints

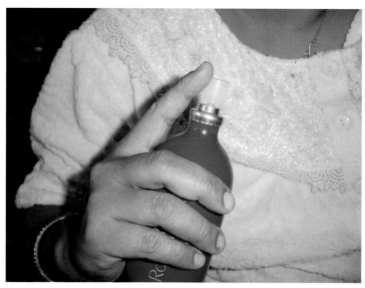

FIGURE 3.19

Due to increased self-image consciousness as well as media advertisements people from all levels of the society are now increasingly addicted to use deodorants and perfumes, especially in spray forms

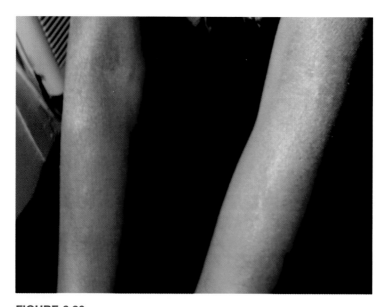

FIGURE 3.20

Airborne contact dermatitis from deodorants affecting the forearms of a lady

4 Investigations of Allergic Contact Dermatitis

PATCH TEST

Principle: to reproduce, in a clinical setting, a mini-model of allergic contact dermatitis using allergens suspended in a vehicle at non-irritant concentration.

> Patch test is the only scientific proof of allergic contact dermatitis
> (Fisher 1986)

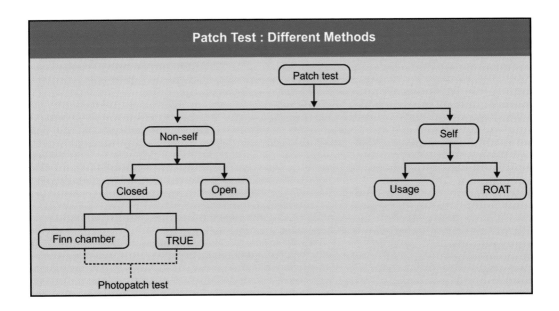

Closed (Non-self) Patch Test [Finn Chamber]

Selection of Patients

1. Taking less than 15 mg of oral steroid (if the patient is on oral steroid therapy)
2. Not applying topical steroid on back for at least 1 week
3. Not having active or flared-up dermatitis
4. Not have been sunburned on back within last 2 weeks
5. Oral antihistamine can be continued during the process.

Indications of Patch Test

1. Allergic Contact Dermatitis Syndrome (ACDS)
2. Atopic dermatitis
3. Nummular dermatitis (nummular eczema)
4. Seborrheic dermatitis (when presenting episodes of acute inflammation)
5. Asteatotic eczema
6. Stasis dermatitis
7. Eczematous lesions around leg ulcer
8. Pompholyx and/or dyshidrotic eczema
9. Lichenification
   [The philosophy behind this strategy is based on the fact that in many cases ACD may supervene upon underlying dermatoses. (Lachapelle and Maibach 2003)]

Instruction to the Patients
(to follow during the patch test procedure)

- Not to take bath or wash or wet the back
- To avoid tight underclothes
- To avoid exercise or activity causing sweating
- To avoid friction/scratching/rubbing on the back
- To avoid strong sun exposure.

Patch Test: Materials

- Finn chambers (shallow aluminium discs to hold allergens)
- Hypoallergenic acrylate tape (Micropore^R)
- Allergens (diluted in various vehicles like petrolatum, water, ethanol, acetone, olive oil, etc.) (In India Indian Standard Battery approved by CODFI [Contact and Occupational Dermatoses Forum of India] is usually employed)
- Marker pen
- Forceps, filter paper discs, cotton, spirit

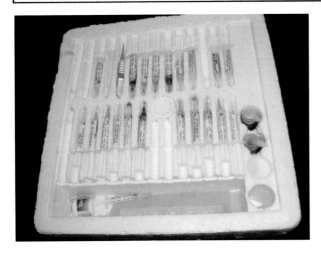

FIGURE 4.1

Allergens kept in the allergen-holding tray with other necessary materials

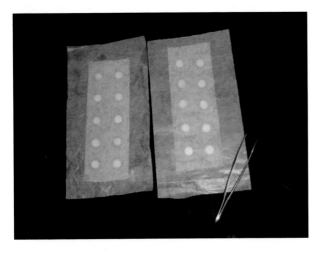

FIGURE 4.2

Finn chambers attached to the protective foil and forceps

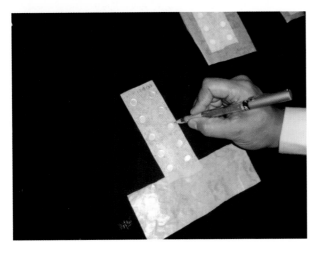

FIGURE 4.3

Finn chambers detached from the protective foil and kept with the aluminium chambers faced up. The protective foil is fixed longitudinally along the edge of the patch test unit

Patch Test: Methods

- Site: upper back (excluding vertebra and scapular angle), deltoid area (for small number of allergens)

- Site should be gently cleansed (with water and alcohol) and dried

- The top of patch test unit is marked and the protective foil removed and they are kept with aluminium chambers faced up

- The protective foil is fixed longitudinally along the edge of the patch test unit to facilitate handling

- 2-3 mm long allergen ointment from the syringe is put at the centre of aluminium chamber to avoid using excess and no allergen should touch the rim of the chambers. In case of liquid antigen a filter paper disc is placed on the Finn chamber by forceps. Then a drop of solution is poured over the filter paper disc.

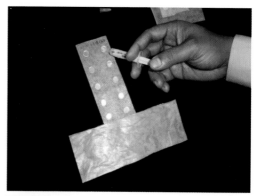

FIGURE 4.4

Allergen from syringe being put on Finn chamber

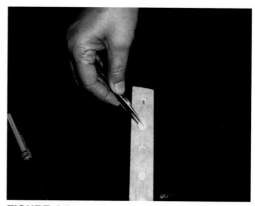

FIGURE 4.5

A filter paper disc being placed on Finn chamber

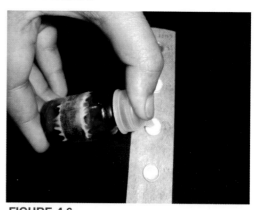

FIGURE 4.6

A drop of liquid allergen being poured over filter paper disc

Patch Test: Methods (Contd.)

- The patch unit is picked up and applied to the back starting from bottom to the top
- Gentle pressure is applied over each chamber to secure better occlusion
- The patches are marked at the corner.

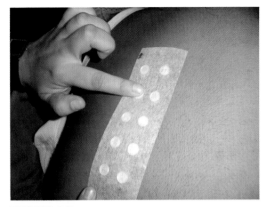

FIGURE 4.7
The patch test unit being applied on the back with gentle pressure on individual chamber

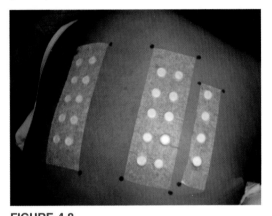

FIGURE 4.8
The patches are marked at the corners

List Of CODFI (Contact and Occupational Dermatoses Forum of India) Allergens [Indian Standard Battery] 2005	
1. Control (petrolatum)	14. Mercaptobenzothiazole
2. Potassium dichromate	15. Nitrofurazone
3. Neomycin sulfate	16. 4-chloro-3-cresol (Chlorocresol)
4. Cobalt chloride-hexahydrate	17. Wool alcohol (Lanolin)
5. Benzocaine	18. Balsam of Peru
6. 4-Phenylenediamine (PPD)	19. Thiuram mix
7. Parabens	20. Chinoform
8. Nickel sulfate-hexahydrate	21. Black rubber mix
9. Colophony	22. P-tert-butylphenol formaldehyde resin
10. Gentamicin sulfate	23. Formaldehyde
11. Mercapto mix	24. Polyethelene Glycol 400
12. Epoxy resin	25. *Parthenium hysterophorus*
13. Fragrance mix	

Patch Test: Readings

Conventionally patch test reading is taken at day 2 (after 48 hours) and again at day 4 (96 hours) (Manuskiatti and Maibach, 1996). In tropical climates where the environmental temperature and humidity are on higher side for most of the year 1-day occlusion may be enough to induce positive patch test response. The shorter occlusion may be more acceptable to the patients and thus may lead to better patients' compliance. Patients are also easily convinced to undergo the patch test procedure (Goh, Wong and Ng, 1994).

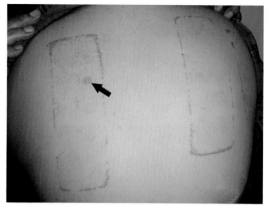

FIGURE 4.9
Positive response after 48 hours (1st reading)

24/48 hours (1st reading)

• The patches are removed and numbered

• The grooves at the sites of the Finn chamber are noted

• Reading are taken 30 minutes after removal of the patch

• The patient is asked not to scratch

72/96 hours (2nd reading)

5/7 Days (3rd reading)

In some cases only (neomycin, corticosteroids).

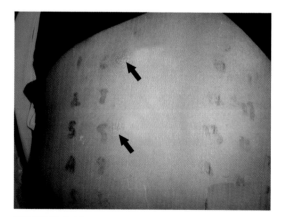

FIGURE 4.10
Positive response after 72 hours (2nd reading)

Patch Test: Analysis

- Current significance (allergen)
- Past significance (allergen)
- Past exposure
- Unknown significance

Patch Test: Interpretation

–	Negative
±	Faint erythema (doubtful)
+	Erythema and papules (non-vesicular)
++	Erythema, papules and vesicles (vesicular)
+++	Erythema, edema and vesicles/bullae/ulceration (bullous/ulceration)
IR	Irritant reaction
NT	Not tested

(After CODFI 2005; Wilkinson et al, 1970 and Ng and Goh, 2001)

Patch Test : Causes of False Reactions

False positive	*False negative*
• Sensitivity to vehicle itself	• Less concentration
• Increased concentration	• Less amount applied
• Impurity (contamination)	• Poor adhesion of patches
• Irritant vehicles	• Inappropriate vehicle
• Excess allergen applied	• Readings seen too early
• Uneven dispersion	• Allergen degraded
• Current or recent dermatitis (at patch site or at distant site)	• Pre-treatment with topical steroid/UV irradiation
• Adhesive tape reaction	• Systemic immuno-suppressant
• Angry back syndrome	
• Edge effect	

[*Angry back syndrome* implies markedly positive patch test response to a particular antigen giving rise to less marked positive responses to antigens at nearby sites.
Edge effects are caused by accumulation of the chemicals at the periphery of the patch test site]

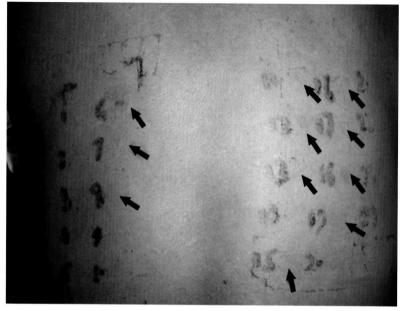

FIGURE 4.11

Allergic sensitivity to vaseline (control) causing false-positive patch test to many allergens which contains vaseline as the vehicle

---

Patch Test: Complications

Generally this is a very safe procedure. Complications are mostly local and reversible.

- Contact dermatitis to 'Micropore' adhesive
- Discomfort from severe reactions (especially when multiple positive severe reactions)
- Flare up of dermatitis
- Angry back syndrome or 'Excited skin syndrome'
- Persistent patch test positive reaction
- Pigmentary changes or keloidal changes
- Rarely: bacterial or viral infection or active sensitization
- Extremely rare: anaphylactoid reaction (especially in contact urticaria).

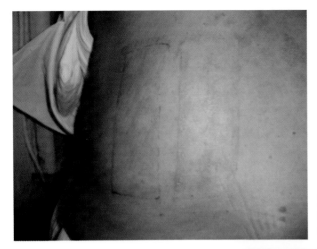

FIGURE 4.12

Contact dermatitis to micropore adhesive showing extensive allergic eruption

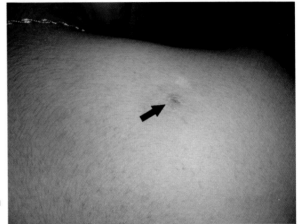

FIGURE 4.13

Persistent patch test reaction even after 6 weeks

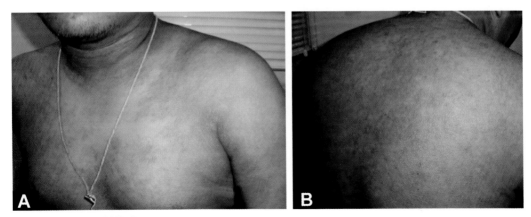

FIGURES 4.14A AND B

Flare up of dermatitis after 1 week following patch test causing generalized erythematous maculopapular eruption

PATCH TEST: OTHER FORMS

Open Patch Test

- The semisolid ointment is put or liquid test substance is dropped on the area of skin measuring about 1 cm in diameter
- In case of solution it is allowed to dry
- The area is kept open, i.e. not covered
- The materials are gently cleansed with dry cotton after 15 to 30 minutes
- Reading is taken after 1 hour; a second reading may be taken after 3/4 days
- Reaction is often weak (may be few isolated papules)
- Indicated in cases of contact urticaria and unknown substances (to avoid anaphylactic reaction)
- A negative open patch test does not preclude that allergy is not present.

Semi-open Test

- In semi-open test the allergens, applied on the skin, are covered by a non-occlusive tape after they have dried off (about 5-10 minutes). This is indicated in industrial or domestic products. The occlusion is done for 2 days and reading is taken at days 2 and 4.

TRUE (Thin Layer Rapid Use Epicutaneous) Test

- Users-friendly, ideal way, ready-to-use patch test system
- Polyester patches coated with allergens in hydrophilic vehicle
- Limitations: cost, limited number of allergens.

ROAT (Repeated Open Application Test)

- The substances are applied twice daily over at least a 5 cm^2 area on upper arm for 7 days
- May help in doubtful positive patch test reactions to preparation in which the suspected allergen is present in a low concentration.

Usage Test

- If patch test becomes negative, the patient is sometimes asked to use the preparation again
- It reproduces the original environment (sweating, friction, damaged skin)
- Cannot differentiate allergic from non-allergic reactions
- Useful in suspected cosmetic and clothing dermatitis.

5 Regional Contact Dermatitis

Regional Assessment: Importance

- Diagnostic clue from the regional location
- Site of location helps in proper and relevant history taking
- Helps to select the allergens to be patch tested.

Face : Common Contactants and Contributory Allergens		
Contactants		*Causative allergens*
Cosmetics	:	Preservative, fragrances
Bindi	:	Glue (PTBP)
Topical medicaments	:	Neomycin, benzyol peroxide
Religious symbol	:	Sandalwood paste
Airborne CD	:	Parthenium, cement dust, spray, deodorants, volatile paints
Contactants in scalp	:	PPD in hair dye
Occupational contact	:	Aerosolized mist (machinist), volatile organic (amine hardener)
Beard-area: after shave, shaving cream	:	Fragrances, balsam of Peru
Photoallergic reaction	:	Oxybenzone, benzophenone

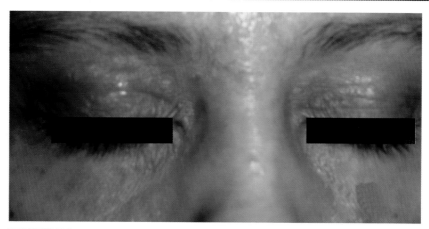

FIGURE 5.1

Eyelid dermatitis of a lady from eye shadows

Eyelids : Common Contactants and Contributory Allergens	
Contactants	*Causative allergens*
Airborne	Parthenium
Cosmetics : nail polish, eye shadows, eye liners, mascara	Formaldehyde resin-varnish
Make-up sponges	Rubber
Topical medications	Neomycin, neosporin, phenylephrine, pilocarpine
Contact lens solution	Preservative
Metal eyelash curlers	Nickel, cobalt, rubber
Occupational (painter)	Acrylates, carnosal

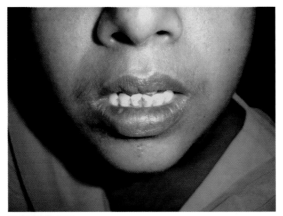

FIGURE 5.2

Contact dermatitis of lip and angle of mouth from lipstick

Lips, Perioral Area, Angle of Mouth: Common Contactants

- Lipstick
- Lipliner
- Lipbalm
- Toothpaste
- Nail polish
- Artificial preservative containing food (parabens)
- Artificially flavored food (containing or cross reacting with balsam of Peru)
- Artificially colored food (azo dye)

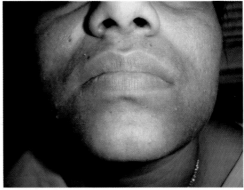

FIGURE 5.3

Perioral contact dermatitis from lipbalm. The patient showed patch positivity to paraben, a preservative of the lipbalm

Intra-oral: Common Contactants

- Dental amalgam
- Dental appliances (nickel, mercury, gold, pallidium)
- Mouth fresheners
- Chewing gum
- Toothpaste
- Oral topical medicaments
- Flavored, preserved or colored food

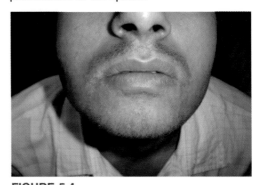

FIGURE 5.4

Perioral contact dermatitis from toothpaste

Scalp : Common Contactants and Contributory Allergens	
Contactants	*Causative allergens*
Hair dye	PPD (paraphenylenediamine)
Shampoos	Fragrances, tar extract, antiseptics
Hair cosmetics	Fragrance, balsam of Peru

Ear: Common Contactants and Contributory Allergens	
Contactants	*Causative allergens*
Ear rings	Nickel, cobalt
Spectacles	Nickel, plastic
Hair dye	PPD (Paraphenylenediamine)
Telephone receiver	Bakelite, phenol formaldehyde resin
Hearing aids	Acrylic
Earphones, earplugs	Plasticizer
Walkman, ipod ear plugs	Acrylic monomer, plasticizer
Topical medicaments	Neosporin, neomycin, gentamycin
Stethoscope ear plug	Rubber

Neck: Common Contactants and Contributory Allergens	
Contactants	*Causative allergens*
Jewellery: Chain, necklace, locket	Nickel, cobalt, exotic woods
Cosmetics: Nail varnish, perfume, after shave lotion	Formaldehyde resin, fragrances
Airborne	Parthenium, ragweed, formaldehyde
Textile	Dye, resin, marking nut extracts
Stethoscope	Metal

Trunk : Common Contactants and Contributory Allergens	
Contactants	*Causative allergens*
Cosmetic : moisturizer, spray, deodorants	Fragrances, preservatives
Airborne	Parthenium, poison ivy
Colored clothing	Azo-aniline dyes
Wrinkle-free clothing	Urea formaldehyde resin
Waistbands (elastic)	Rubber allergens
Spandex bras	Rubber allergens
Buttons, belt buckles, safety pins, key chain	Nickel, cobalt
Topical medicaments	Neomycin, neosporin

Axillae: Common Sites and Contactants		
Sites		*Contactants*
Axillary vault	:	Deodorant, perfume
Axillary folds	:	Textile

HAND DERMATITIS

Hand represents a very common site for both irritant and allergic contact dermatitis. Sometimes both types persist simultaneously.

Housewives dermatitis and occupational contact dermatitis predominantly involve hands.

Common Causes of Hand Dermatitis

- Soaps and detergent (more commonly irritant contact dermatitis)
- Foods and spices
- Industrial solvents and oils
- Cement
- Metal
- Topical medicaments
- Rubber gloves
- Purse
- Bags, briefcase
- Bike, scooter
- Sports material (Cricket bat, tennis racket)

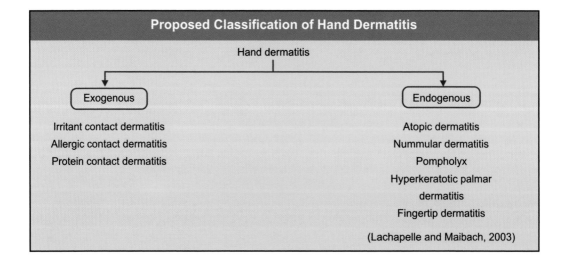

Proposed Classification of Hand Dermatitis

Hand dermatitis

Exogenous

Irritant contact dermatitis
Allergic contact dermatitis
Protein contact dermatitis

Endogenous

Atopic dermatitis
Nummular dermatitis
Pompholyx
Hyperkeratotic palmar
dermatitis
Fingertip dermatitis

(Lachapelle and Maibach, 2003)

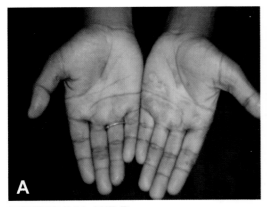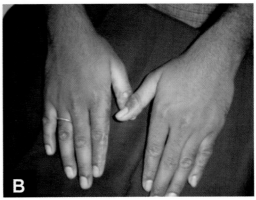

FIGURES 5.5A AND B

Allergic contact dermatitis from rubber gloves in a health care personnel

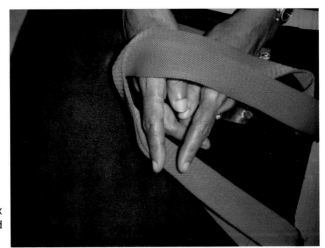

FIGURE 5.6

Allergic contact dermatitis of index fingers from contact with bags colored with azo dye

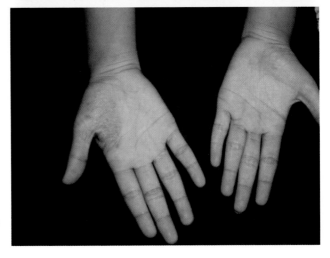

FIGURE 5.7

Allergic contact dermatitis from the steering cover of the car

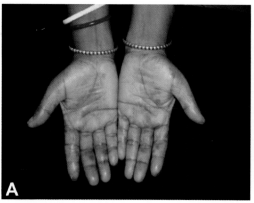 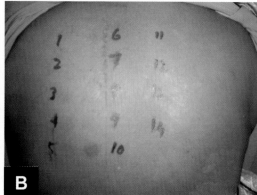

FIGURES 5.8A AND B

Allergic contact dermatitis of hands of a lady who showed patch test positivity to garlic

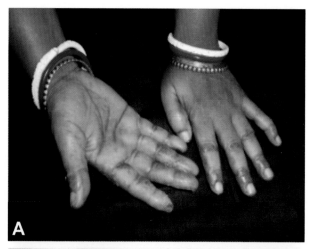

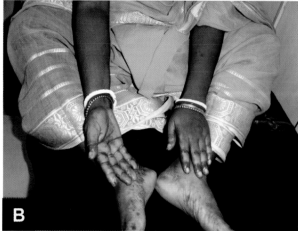

FIGURES 5.9A AND B

Cumulative irritant contact dermatitis of hands and feet from detergent and liquid soap

Vesicular Hand Dermatitis

Vesicular hand dermatitis or 'pompholyx' type eruption represents a unique type of hand dermatitis showing recurrent vesicular eruption at the sides of fingers followed by scaling.

Causes of Vesicular Hand Dermatitis

- Secondary 'ide' eruption to primary contact dermatitis elsewhere in the body (feet)
- Secondary 'ide' eruption to fungus eruption elsewhere in the body (groin, feet, etc.)
- Systemic reactivation of contact dermatitis (e.g. Nickel sensitivity)
- Idiopathic

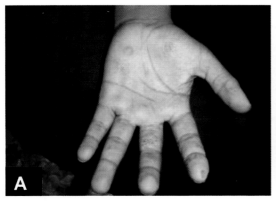
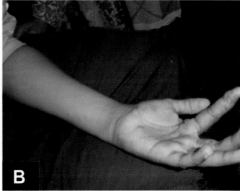

FIGURES 5.10A and B

Vesicular hand dermatitis of a boy who showed strongly positive nickel sensitivity in patch test reaction

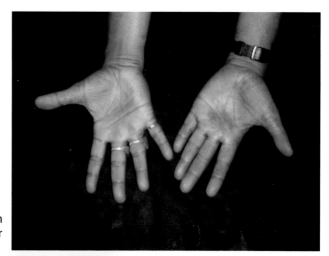

FIGURE 5.11

Allergic contact dermatitis from industrial solvents in a factory worker

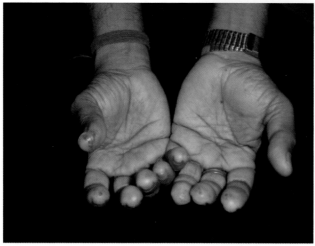

FIGURE 5.12

Fingertip dermatitis of a priest by handling the flower 'tagar' *(Ervatamia coronaria)*

Fingertip Dermatitis in Different Occupations: Common Contactants and Contributory Allergens		
Occupation	*Contactants*	*Causative allergens*
Hair dressing	Permanent hair straightening solution	Glyceryl monothioglycolate
	Hair dye	PPD
Nursery	Disinfectants	Glutaraldehyde
Dental and orthopedic surgery	Glue	Methacrylates
Housewives	Detergent Vegetables, flowers, sandalwood paste	

Arms and Forearms: Common Contactants

- Mostly by same contactants as of hands
- Bangles, watch and watchbands (leather, metal)
- Amulet ('Maduli')
- Amulet string or chain
- Soap and moisturizer
- Deodorant, perfumes
- Industrial chemical and solvents
- Plants

Anogenital Area : Common Contactants and Causative Allergens

Contactants	Causative allergens
Contraception devices	Rubber
Soap and sanitary pads	Antiseptics, fragrance, balsam of Peru
Topical medicaments	Local anesthetics, ointment bases and emulsifiers, antibiotics
Toilet paper	Dyes and perfume
Toilet seats	Rubber, acrylic polymer
Occupational allergens	

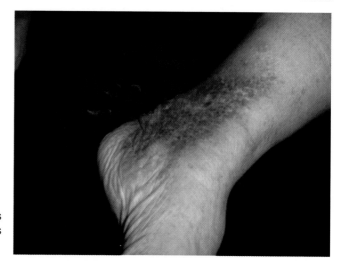

FIGURE 5.13

Stasis dermatitis on lower legs caused secondary contact dermatitis by application of topical neomycin

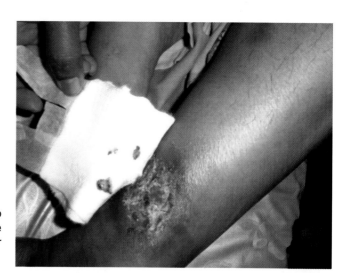

FIGURE 5.14

Stasis ulcer in lower leg had led to surrounding contact dermatitis by the topical antiseptics (Dettol) used for dressing

Thighs and Lower Legs: Contactants and Contributory Allergens	
Contactants	*Causative allergens*
Clothing	Coloring materials
Pantry hose	Dye
Topical medicaments	Benzocaine, neomycin, lanolin, parabens
Cosmetics, moisturizers	Preservatives, vehicles, fragrances
Rubber boots and socks	Rubber compound
Socks	Color
Stasis dermatitis/ulcer	Topical medicaments

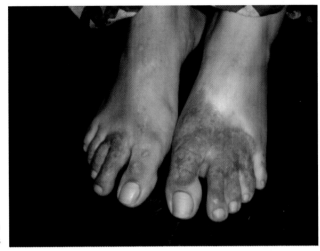

FIGURE 5.15

Allergic contact dermatitis on dorsum of both feet induced by rubber sandals

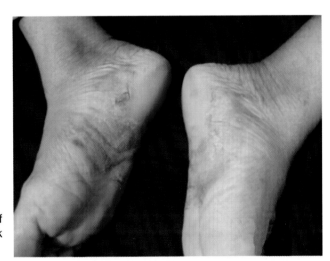

FIGURE 5.16

Allergic contact dermatitis on sole of feet of a mason who used to do work with wet cement in bare feet

Feet : Common Contactants and Contributory Allergens	
Contactants	*Allergens*
Shoe	Glue: Paratertiary butylphenol formaldehyde resin (PTBP) Rubber components Chromate (used to tan leather) Metal (Nickel)
Cement	Chromate, cobalt
Topical medicines	Neomycin, neosporin, adhesive plaster, miconazole, econazole

6

Non-Eczematous Contact Dermatitis

Contact dermatitis sometimes do not present clinical features of classic eczematous dermatitis. Instead they manifest as different morphological pattern of eruption other than eczema.

Non-Eczematous Contact Dermatitis
- Lichenoid contact dermatitis
- Pigmented contact dermatitis
- Bullous contact dermatitis
- Purpuric contact dermatitis
- Erythema multiforme like contact dermatitis
- Contact urticaria

LICHENOID CONTACT DERMATITIS OR LICHEN PLANUS-LIKE CD

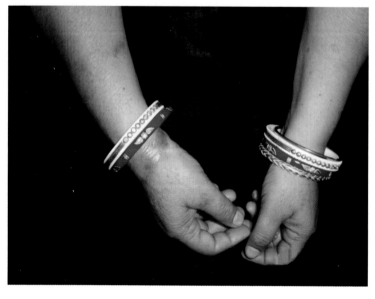

FIGURE 6.1
Lichenoid contact dermatitis induced by the red dye of the bangles used by the lady

Lichenoid contact dermatitis or lichen planus like contact dermatitis denotes skin eruption morphologically similar to lichen planus induced by various chemicals.

Clinically the lesions may mimick classic lichen planus but the papules are usually larger and scaly and Wickham's striae are usually absent. Post-inflammatory hyperpigmentation is more pronounced in lichenoid CD than classic LP. Mucous membrane is involved less commonly.

Sometimes the lichenoid CD may be generalized producing eczematous papules, plaques and variable desquamation.

Histopathologically classic LP and lichenoid CD are often similar. Lichenoid CD may have some special features:

- Focal parakeratosis
- Focal hypogranulosis
- Greater amount of spongiosis
- Larger number of necrotic keratino-cytes and cytoid bodies
- More pleomorphic cellular infiltrate
- Plenty plasma cells and eosinophils
- Deeper perivascular infiltrate
- Less dense lymphocytic infiltrate; not band-like

Lichenoid CD: Common Contributory Agents

1. Color film processing chemicals
   - Substituted para-phenylene diamine PPD-A
2. Socks and shoes color
   - Paraphenylenediamine (PPD)
3. Cosmetic
   - Musk ambrette
4. Temporary tattos
   - PPD
   - Commercial black henna
5. Red ink/color
   - Azo dye
6. Automobile
   - Methacrylic acid esters
7. Health personnel
   - Aminoglycoside antibiotic
   - Chlorpheniramine maleate
8. Metals
   - Nickel
   - Mercury
   - Silver
   - Gold

Oral Lichenoid CD: Common Contributory Agents

1. Dental fillers/restorative devices
   - Methacrylic acid ester
   - Silver
   - Gold
   - Mercury
2. Balsam of Peru
3. Fragrances
   - Cinnamic aldehyde

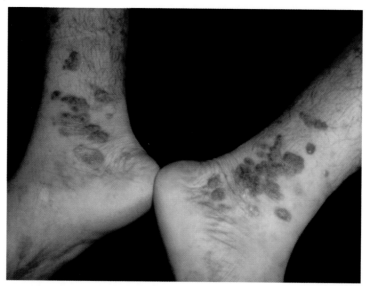

FIGURE 6.2

Lichenoid contact dermatitis localized to lower legs for 2 years originating from socks color (black containing PPD). The patient had no other features of lichen planus elsewhere in the body including oral mucosa

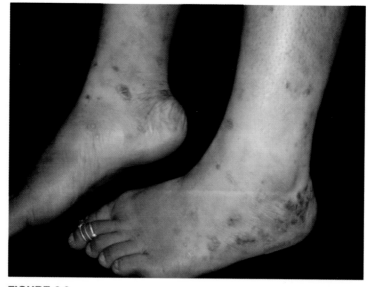

FIGURE 6.3

Lichenoid contact dermatitis of feet and lower legs induced by black shoes containing PPD

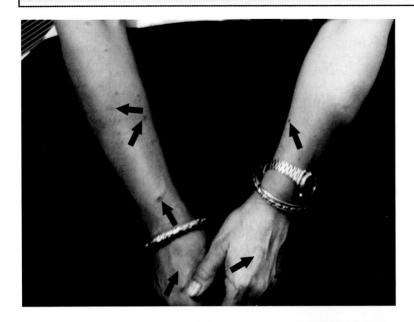

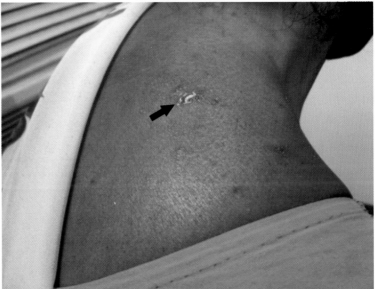

FIGURES 6.4 and 6.5
Lichenoid CD on the forearm and back of the lady caused by the fabric paint and glass paint in her professional use as a designer. Patch test showed positivity to PPD and cobalt.

ORAL LICHENOID CONTACT DERMATITIS

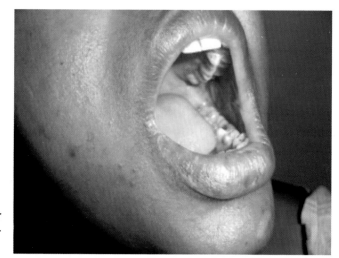

FIGURE 6.6

Oral lichenoid contact dermatitis over the buccal mucosa caused by long-standing dental filling

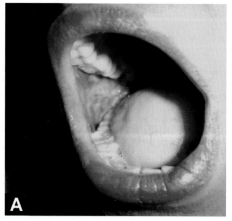

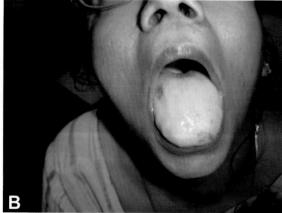

FIGURES 6.7A AND B

Oral lichenoid contact dermatitis in a lady on buccal mucosa as well as tongue caused by clove (balsam of Peru) repeatedly being sucked as mouth freshener

PIGMENTED CONTACT DERMATITIS

Pigmented contact dermatitis represents clinical features of hyperpigmentation produced by chemicals without having any preceding itching or eczema.

Patch test shows either an eczematous eruption or a hyperpigmented patch.

Pigmented contact dermatitis is more common in oriental population.

> **Pigmented Contact Dermatitis: Common Offending Agents**
> 1. Washing agents
>   - Optical whitener
> 2. Cosmetics
>   - Pigments (D and C Yellow/Red)
>   - Jasmine oil
>   - Rose oil
>   - Musk ambrette
> 3. Ornament
>   - Bindi (Kumkum) [Sudan 1]
> 4. Textile
>   - Naphthol AS (dye)
>   - Azo dye
>   - Coupling agents

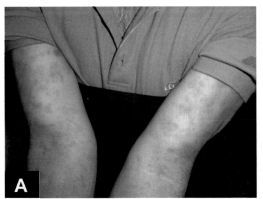 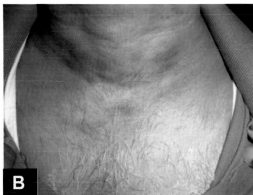

FIGURES 6.8A AND B

Pigmented contact dermatitis on both forearms, neck and V-area of chest caused by fragrances of deodorant containing musk ambrette

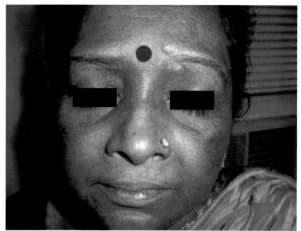

FIGURE 6.9

Pigmented contact dermatitis of a lady on the face induced by some cosmetics containing pigments

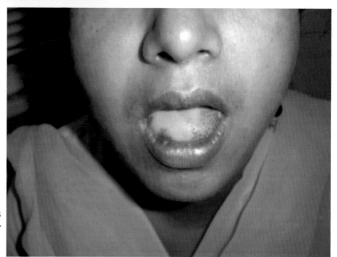

FIGURE 6.10

Pigmented contact dermatitis of lips and front part of the tongue by color of the lipstick (Sudan 1)

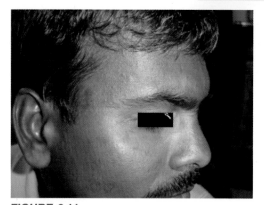

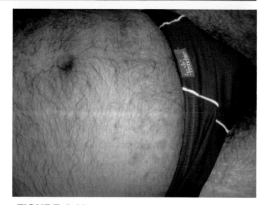

FIGURE 6.11

Pigmented contact dermatitis of face in a textile worker who had to expose to azo dyes

FIGURE 6.12

Pigment contact dermatitis on lower abdomen caused by textile dye (azo dye) of jangia

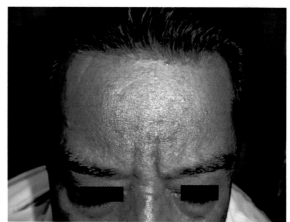

FIGURE 6.13

Pigmented contact dermatitis of a person on the forehead developed by his obsessive use of fragrance containing musk ambrette

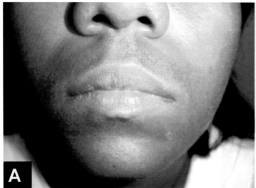

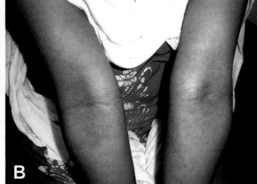

FIGURES 6.14A AND B

Pigmented contact dermatitis of a young girl aged 18 years especially around her lips and forearms developed from the use of a moisturizing cream containing paraben as preservative

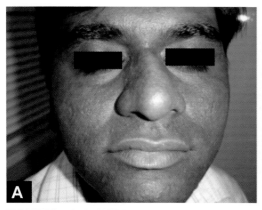

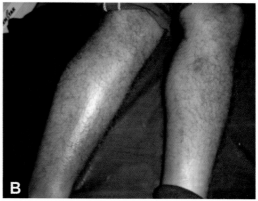

FIGURES 6.15A AND B

Pigmented CD of a person on face as well as both legs by the use of hair dye (PPD) on scalp and black socks containing PPD. Patch test showed strong positivity to PPD

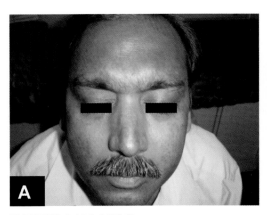
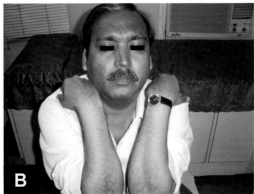

FIGURES 6.16A AND B

Pigment contact dermatitis over the forehead and forearms developed in a textile engineer who was in regular exposure to azo dye and coupling agents used in that industry

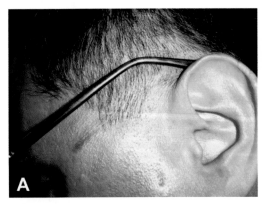
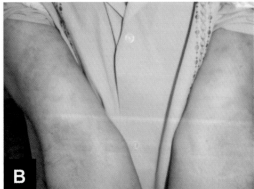

FIGURES 6.17A AND B

Pigmented contact dermatitis in a same person by using a spectacle frame containing azo dye and over the forearm from use of fragrance (rose oil and jasmine oil)

BULLOUS CONTACT DERMATITIS

Bullous contact dermatitis produces bullous eruption clinically and histologically similar to bullous pemphigoid. However, the lesions are usually localized. Direct immunofluorescence testing shows negative result.

Bullous Contact Dermatitis: Contributory Allergens

- Cinnamon powder
- Cinnamaldehyde
- Cinnamic alcohol
- Potassium dichromate
- Nickel

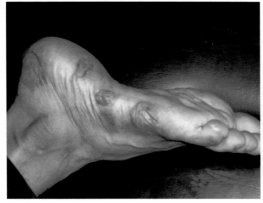

FIGURE 6.18

Bullous contact dermatitis localised to feet caused by potassium dichromate used in processing of leather. Patch test showed strong positivity to potassium dichromates

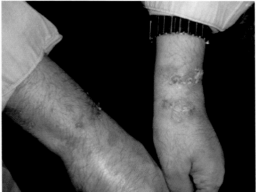

FIGURE 6.19

Bullous contact dermatitis localised to both wrists caused by the metal wrist-band used by him in both wrists by rotation. Patch test showed positive nickel sensitivity

PURPURIC CONTACT DERMATITIS

Purpuric contact dermatitis is mostly allergic in origin. Some may, however, be irritant in nature.

Purpuric CD: Causes

1. Shoes, sandals
   - Antioxidant in black rubber (subsitituted PPD)
2. Textile dyes
   - Navy blue uniform (azodye, Disperse Blue 85)
3. Topical drugs
   - Topical NSAID
   - Proflavine

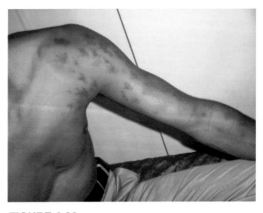

FIGURE 6.20
Purpuric contact dermatitis caused by wearing navy blue uniform containing dye (Disperse Blue 85)

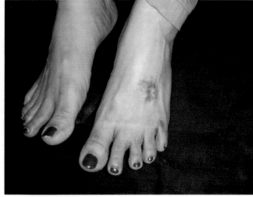

FIGURE 6.21
Purpuric contact dermatitis induced by topical pain-relieving agent used for sprain

ERYTHEMA MULTIFORME-LIKE CONTACT DERMATITIS

Features

- The morphology of the lesions at the point of origin is usually eczematous
- Peripheral-most lesion spreading at distant may be erythema-multiforme like target lesion. In between the eczematous lesion at the site of origin and peripheral-most erythema multiforme lesions there could be various morphological pattern of lesions like papules, plaques and urticaria
- Lesions are usually limited
- Histopathology, not showing features of classic erythema multiforme, can be non-specific in nature
- Patch test positive response shows eczematous reaction.

Erythema Multiforme: Causative Allergens

1. Plants
   - Mango, poison ivy
2. Topical woods
   - Brazilian rosewood
3. Topical medicaments
   - Proflavine
   - Vitamin E
   - Topical corticosteroid
   - Vioform
4. Epoxy resin

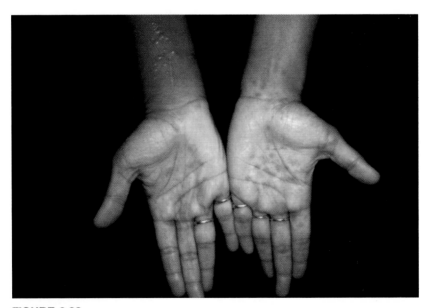

FIGURE 6.22

Erythema multiforme like eruption on palms spreading from the primary site of acute contact dermatitis (eczematous) of the wrist

CONTACT URTICARIA

Contact urticaria syndrome was first described by Maibach and Johnson (1975).

Urticarial lesions develop instantly on direct exposure to the offending substance.

Clinically the lesions are like classical urticaria having wheals and flare. In atopics, the existing eczematous patches are exacerbated without producing any wheals causing difficulty in diagnosis. Systemic symptoms can be seen in contact urticaria like rhinitis, conjunctivitis, dyspnea and even shock (anaphylactoid reactions).

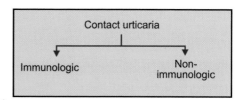

Diagnosis of Contact Urticaria

- Detailed history
- Skin testing
  - Open patch test
  - Prick test
  - Scratch test

Natural rubber latex (NRL) is a common cause of contact urticaria. Cross-reaction with NRL has been seen with banana (latex-banana syndrome), chestnut and avocado.

Non-immunologic Contact Urticaria: Common Causes		
Fragrance and flavor	*Animals*	*Preservatives/Germicidals*
Balsam of Peru	Caterpillars	Sodium benzoate
Cinnamic acid	Arthropods	Benzoic Acid
Vanilla	Jellyfish	Formaldehyde
Menthol		Chlorocresol
	Medicines	
Foods	Benzocaine	*Plants*
Fish	Alcohol	Chrysanthemum
Prawn	Capsaicin	Miscellaneous
Crab	Camphor	Cobalt chloride
Capsicum	Methyl salicylate	Resorcinol
		Turpentine

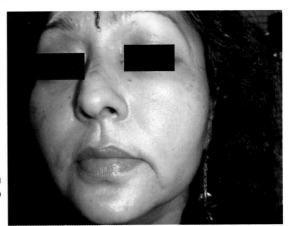

FIGURE 6.23

The lady developed acute contact urticaria on both cheeks after applying a make-up containing balsam of Peru

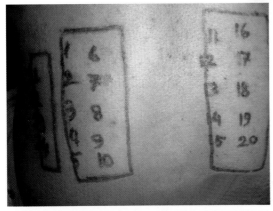

FIGURE 6.24

Open patch test showing positivity to parabens

Immunologic Contact Urticaria : Common Causes		
Fragrances and flavoring agents	*Medicines*	*Preservatives*
Balsam of Peru	Acetylsalicylic acid	Formaldehyde
Cinnamic aldehyde	Ampicillin	Benzoic acid
Benzoic acid	Bacitracin	Parabens
Menthol	Benzocaine	
Vanillin	Benzoyl peroxide	*Miscellaneous*
	Penicillin	Acrylic monomer
Food	Lindane	Ammonium persulfate
Egg		Epoxy resin
Banana	*Metals*	Formaldehyde resin
Tortoise	Nickel	Hypochlorite
Prawn	Cobalt	Naphtha
Crab		Nylon
Garlic	*Plants*	Polyethylene glycol
Brinjal	Chrysanthemum	Plastic
	Colophony	Potassium ferricyanide
Hair cosmetics	Garlic	Textile finish
Henna	Latex rubber	Xylene
PPD	Papain	
Potassium persulfate		

7

Contact Dermatitis from Topical Medicaments

Contact dermatitis, both irritant and allergic types, from topical medicaments are fairly common in daily practice. About one third of all cases of contact dermatitis are initiated or perpetuated by topical medicaments.

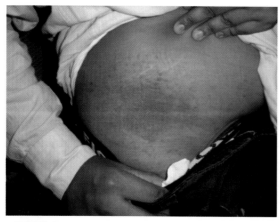

FIGURE 7.1

Irritant contact dermatitis from 'Dettol' (chloroxylenol) on abdominal skin after application over an insect allergy.

Topical Medicaments : Common Causes of Contact Dermatitis

A. *Antibacterial agents/Antibiotics*
　1. Nitrofurazone
　2. Neomycin
　3. Framycetin
　4. Gentamycin
　5. Bacitracin
　6. Polymyxin
　7. Acriflavine
　8. Proflovine

B. *Antiseptics/Preservatives*
　1. Cetrimide
　2. Benzalkonium chloride
　3. Ammoniated mercury
　4. Mercurochrome
　5. Thiomerosal
　6. Chlorhexidine
　7. Hexachlorophene
　8. Chloroxylenol
　9. Chlorocresol
　10. Parabens
　11. Kathon CG
　12. Quaternium 15
　13. Formaldehyde

C. *Local Anesthetic*
　1. Benzocaine

D. *Antihistamines*
　1. Phenothiazines
　2. Ethylenediamines

E. *Bases*
　1. Propylene glycol
　2. Polyethylene glycol
　3. Lanolin
　4. Petrolatum

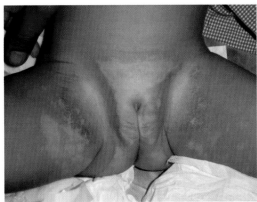

FIGURE 7.2

Irritant contact dermatitis from regular use of 'Savlon' for washing the genital area of the infant skin

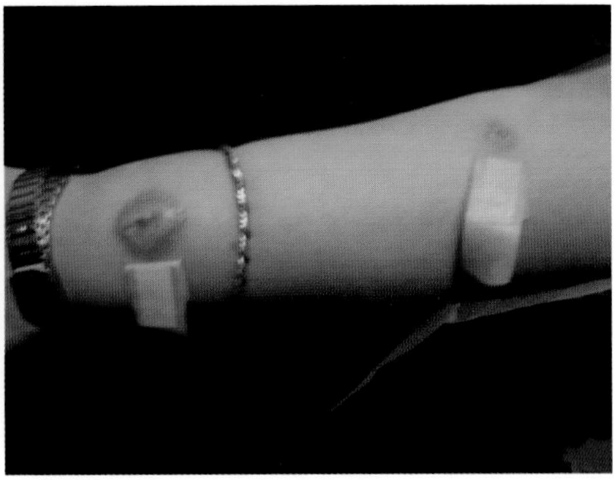

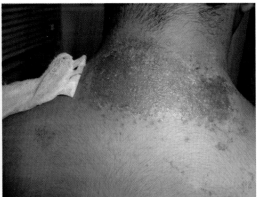

FIGURE 7.3

Allergic contact dermatitis from mercurochrome used in 'Band-aid' plaster

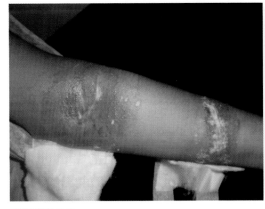

FIGURE 7.4

Allergic contact dermatitis from neomycin used as antiseptic for a wound

FIGURE 7.5

Allergic contact dermatitis from soframycin (framycetin) used upon a wound

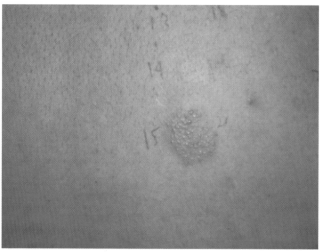

FIGURE 7.6
Patch test shows strong positivity to 'nitrofurazone'

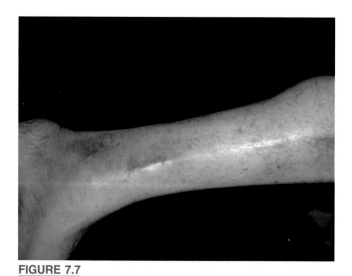

FIGURE 7.7
Allergic contact dermatitis on lower legs at the donor site of coronary arterial by-pass operation, while applying some medicaments containing lanolin

8 Contact Dermatitis from Footwear

Footwear dermatitis remains one of the most common forms of contact dermatitis. In India this represents a distinct group of all contact dermatitis (Bajaj, 1988)

For constant change in the fashions, the manufacturers are regularly changing their design and the materials. The closed environment inside a shoe especially in hot and humid climate along with various types of chemicals of shoes provide an ideal milieu for development of shoe dermatitis.

A secondary 'ide eruption', i.e. vesicular dermatitis on the hands is occasionally seen in shoe dermatitis. Wearing shoes with the help of hands can also lead to contact of shoe chemicals on hands. Sites other than hands are also sometimes associated with shoe dermatitis.

Chemicals of Footwear: Cause of Contact Dermatitis

Shoes
A. Tanning of leather
   1. Chromium compound
   2. Formaldehyde
B. Rubber
   1. Mercaptobenzothiazole
   2. Tetramethylthiuram disulfide
C. Adhesive
   1. Para-tertiarybutyl phenol formaldehyde resin (PTBP)
   2. Colophony (in shoe cement)
D. Plastic
   1. Bisphenol A
E. Color
   1. Parephenylenediamine (PPD)
   2. Azo dye

Socks
A. Inner lining
   1. Latex adhesive
   2. Thiuram
   3. Mercaptobenzothiazole
B. Color
   1. PPD (Saha and Srinivas, 1985)
   2. Azo dyes

The constituents of leather, rubber, metals, color and adhesives are the most common cause of shoe allergic contact dermatitis.
(Chowdhuri and Ghosh, 2007)

Contact Dermatitis from Leather Shoes

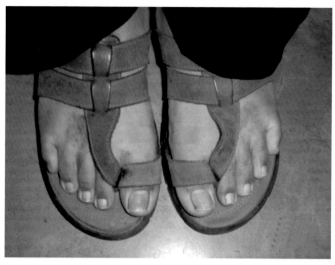

FIGURE 8.1

Contact dermatitis from leather shoes; patch test showed potassium dichromate positivity

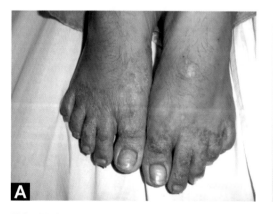

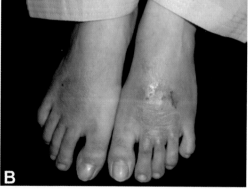

FIGURES 8.2A AND B

Contact dermatitis from leather shoes showing patch test positivity to chromate

Contact Dermatitis from Rubber Shoes

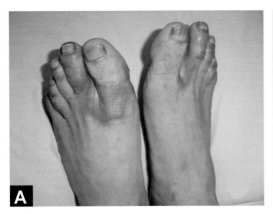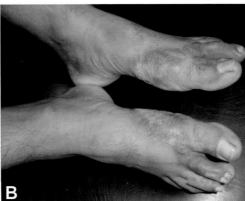

FIGURES 8.3A AND B
Contact dermatitis from rubber shoe; patch test showed positivity to mercaptobenzothiazole

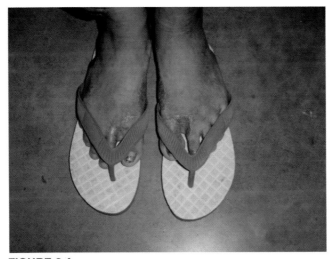

FIGURE 8.4
Contact dermatitis from rubber chappal; patch test showed positivity to tetramethylthiuram disulfide

Contact Dermatitis from Shoe Adhesive

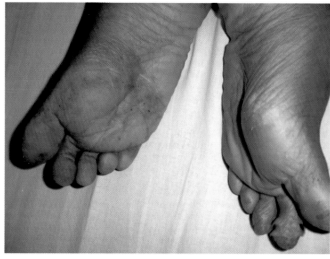

FIGURE 8.5
Contact dermatitis from shoe adhesive; patch test showed positivity to PTBPFR (Para-tertiary butyl phenol formaldehyde resin)

Contact Dermatitis from Socks

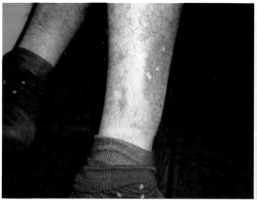

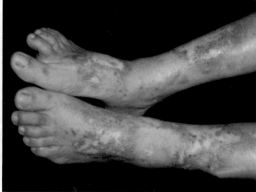

FIGURE 8.6
Allergic contact dermatitis from elastic lining of the socks having patch test positivity to thiuram

FIGURE 8.7
Allergic contact dermatitis from synthetic socks showing positive patch test to mercaptobenzothiazole

Contact Dermatitis from Shoe/Socks Color

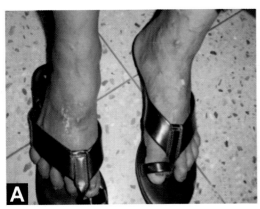

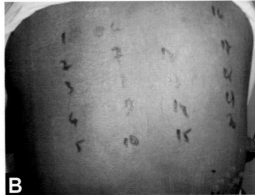

FIGURES 8.8A AND B
Contact dermatitis from black color of chappal showing patch positivity to PPD

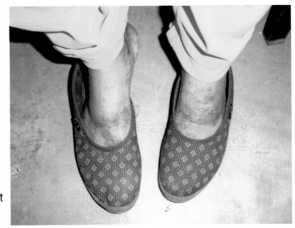

FIGURE 8.9
Contact dermatitis from shoe color; patient showed positive patch response to PPD

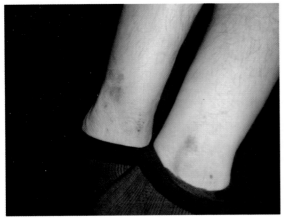

FIGURE 8.10
Contact dermatitis from color of socks; the patient showed positive patch response to PPD

Footwear Dermatitis causing Secondary 'Ide' Eruptions

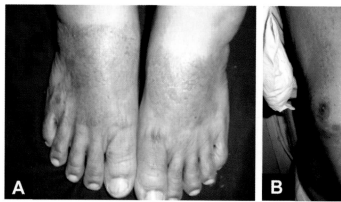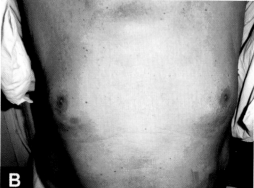

FIGURES 8.11A AND B

Allergic contact dermatitis of feet from chromate of leather causing 'ide eruption' on the trunk

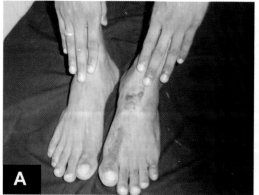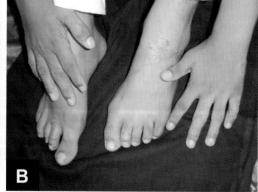

FIGURES 8.12A AND B

Allergic contact dermatitis of two different patients from footwear on feet having patch positivity to potassium dichromate showing also hand dermatitis from secondary 'ide eruptions'

9 Contact Dermatitis from Cosmetics

About 4% of patients routinely patch tested for contact dermatitis react to cosmetic.

Recently extensive use of cosmetics in all socio-economic classes has caused alarming rise in the incidence of contact dermatitis from cosmetics.

Fragrances, parabens and lanolin showed 25.8%, 36.3% and 7.9% respectively among routinely patch tested patients (Sen, Mukhopadhyaya, Ghosh, IAISD, 2006).

Cosmetic Dermatitis : Features

- Cosmetic dermatitis predominantly affects the females
- Face most commonly involved
- Types of reaction:
  (a) Irritant contact
  (b) Allergic contact
  (c) Photo contact
  (d) Contact urticaria

Cosmetic Dermatitis: Commonest Cause

- Fragrance ingredients
- Preservative
- PPD (P-paraphenylene diamine)
- Lanolin derivative
- Glycerine thioglycolate
- Formaldehyde resin
- Sunscreen and other UV absorber
- Methacrylate

Cosmetics : Important Contact Sensitizers		
Cosmetic group	*Cosmetic*	*Common sensitizers*
Hair cosmetic	Hair dye	PPD
	Shaving solution	Thioglycolate
	Shampoo	Detergent base, sodium lauryl ether sulfate
Facial cosmetics	Perfumes	Fragrances
	Lipstick	Eosin, azodye, carmin
	Bindi	Coat tar, PVC, adhesive (PTBP)
Eye cosmetic	Eye shadow	Paraben, colophony
Nail cosmetic	Varnish	Resin
	Artificial	Methacrylate
	Hardener	Formaldehyde

Contact Dermatitis from Hair Dye (PPD)

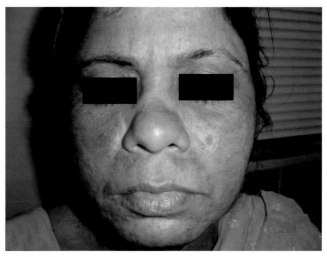

FIGURE 9.1
Hair dye affecting a lady on her face; patch test showed strong positive result to PPD

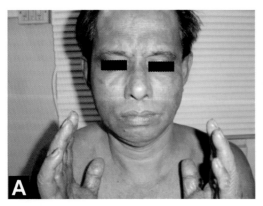
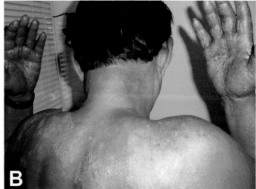

FIGURE 9.2A AND B
Hair dye allergy in a man affecting face, trunk and limbs. Patch test showed positive result to PPD

Contact Dermatitis from Bindi

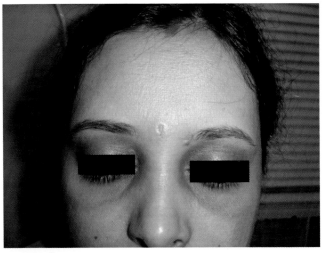

FIGURE 9.3
Bindi dermatitis in a lady after using 'bindi'. Patch test showed positivity to PTBP

Contact Dermatitis from Lip Cosmetics

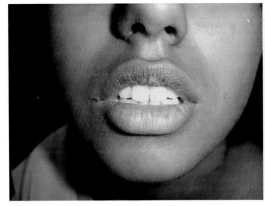 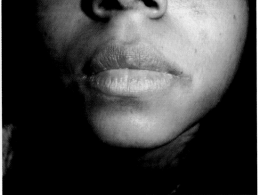

FIGURE 9.4
Contact cheilitis from use of lipstick; patch test positivity was seen to parabens

FIGURE 9.5
Contact cheilitis from use of lipgloss. Patch test showed positive response to formaldehyde

Contact Dermatitis from Shaving Cream

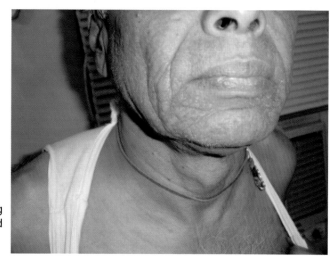

FIGURE 9.6

Contact dermatitis of a man affecting beard area, Patch test showed positive response to fragrance mix

Contact Dermatitis from Nail Polish

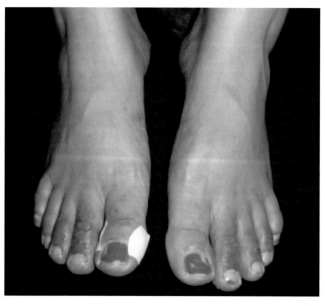

FIGURE 9.7

Contact dermatitis from nail polish. Patch test positive response was seen to resin

10 Contact Dermatitis from Ornaments

Contact dermatitis from the ornaments used for the decorative purpose of body is fairly common. The common offending agents metal (nickel, cobalt), plastics (epoxy resins, phenol formaldehyde), glues and adhesives (formaldehyde resins), coloring metals (PPD, azodyes) of the ornaments may cause different types of contact dermatitis.

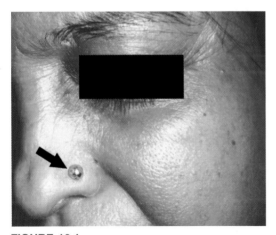

FIGURE 10.1

Contact dermatitis of nose from nose-ring containing nickel

Different Ornaments causing Contact Dermatitis

Head and scalp
- Hair band

Forehead
- Forehead-chain

Nose
- Nose ring

Ears
- Ear ring

Neck
- Necklace
- Chain

Arms
- Arm chain
- Amulet-holding chain/string

Chest
- Chain
- Locket

Wrist
- Wrist band
- Bangles
- Wrist-watch

Waist
- Chain
- Amulet-holding chain/string

Legs
- Chain

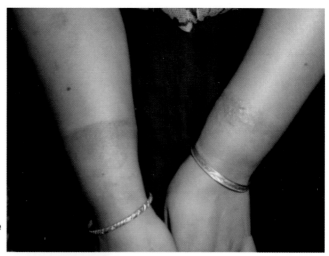

FIGURE 10.2
Contact dermatitis from bangles made
of nickel on the wrist of a lady

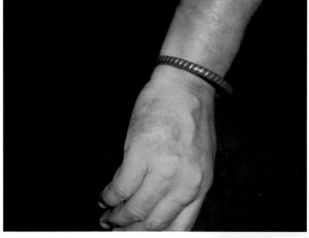

FIGURE 10.3
Contact dermatitis from bangle (plastic)
on the hand

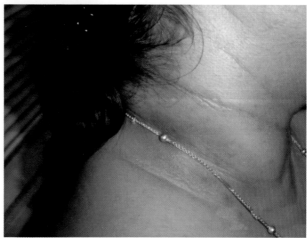

FIGURE 10.4
Contact dermatitis on neck from a nickel-
containing chain

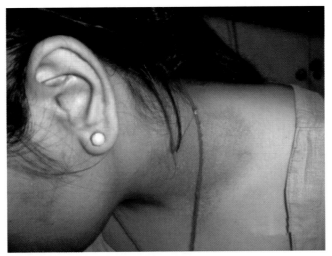

FIGURE 10.5

Contact dermatitis on neck from the red color (azo dye) of the string used on the neck to hold amulet

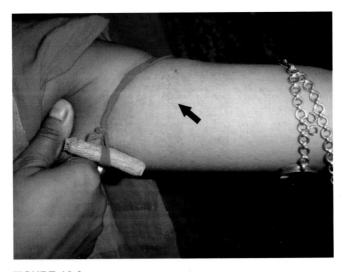

FIGURE 10.6

Contact dermatitis of the arm from the red color (azo dye) of the string holding a root-amulet. She had a silver chain on the same arm without producing any dermatitis.

11 Contact Dermatitis from Daily-Usage Objects

Contact dermatitis from the daily-usage materials are also quite common. These objects are endless in number and varieties, especially in this new era of consumer explosion. In developing countries these are particularly prevalent as people while using some cheaper brands get exposure to more allergenic materials. Quality control of these products are often not ensured.

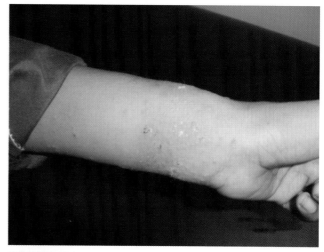

FIGURE 11.1
Contact dermatitis of the wrist from the wrist watch band

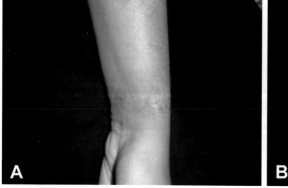

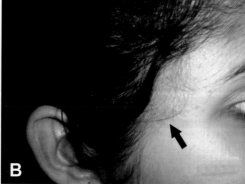

FIGURES 11.2A AND B
Contact dermatitis of the wrist from the wrist watch band and face from the spectacle frame in the same patient – both caused by nickel

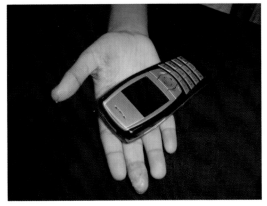

FIGURE 11.3

Contact dermatitis of fingers and palm from using mobile phone (nickel)

FIGURE 11.4

Contact dermatitis of hand from using purse (leather)

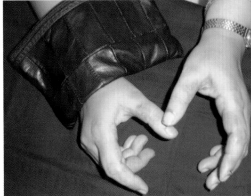

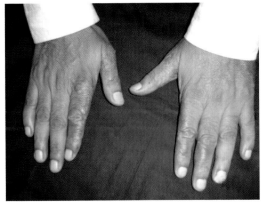

FIGURE 11.5

Contact dermatitis of hands caused by holding briefcase

FIGURE 11.6

Contact dermatitis of left leg from the nickel screw of the artificial support of the right leg

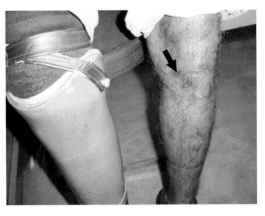

12 Occupational Contact Dermatitis

- About 30% of occupational injury and 40% of occupational diseases are dermatological in origin.
- About 90% of occupational skin diseases are contact dermatitis among which majority are irritant in nature
- Hands remain the most commonly affected site of occupational dermatoses.

Predisposing Factors of Occupational Dermatoses

Host related
- Atopic dermatitis
- Psoriasis
- Acne
- Systemic diseases
- Stasis
- Skin color
- Hygiene

Job related
- Irritants
- Allergens
- Infections
- Carcinogens

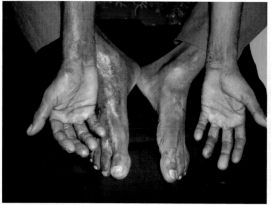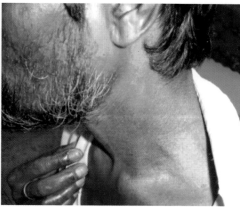

FIGURE 12.1

Contact dermatitis of hands, feet and neck of a mason who uses cement for construction (patch test showed positivity to potassium dichromate)

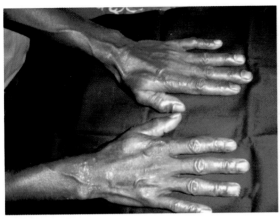
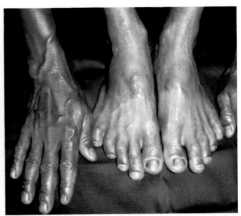

FIGURE 12.2

Contact dermatitis of both hands and feet of a helper in the construction works from cement. Patch test positivity was seen with chromates

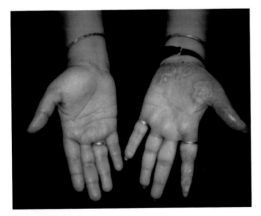
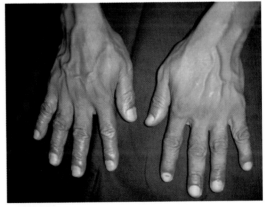

FIGURE 12.3

Occupational contact dermatitis on hands of a lady, who is a textile designer, from the azo dyes of the textiles

FIGURE 12.4

Occupational contact dermatitis of a 'phoochka (water-balls)-seller' from the use of various vegetables and tasty salts

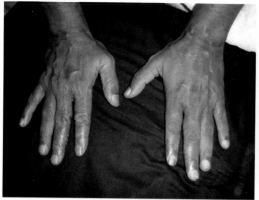

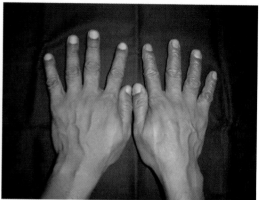

FIGURE 12.5

Occupational contact dermatitis of a farmer on his hands from the rice dust containing pesticides

FIGURE 12.6

Occupational contact dermatitis on the hands of a farmer from the fertilizers used in the agriculture works

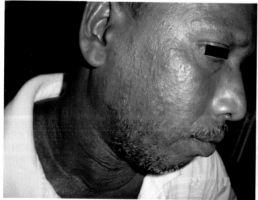

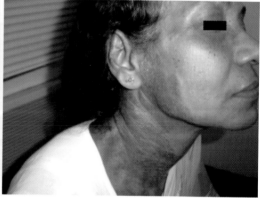

FIGURE 12.7

Occupational airborne contact dermatitis of a newspaper seller from the paper dust

FIGURE 12.8

Occupational airborne contact dermatitis of a painter who used acrylic paint in spray form

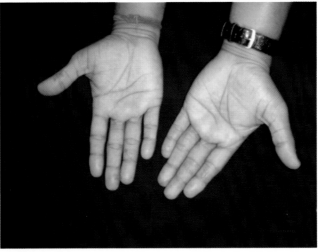

FIGURE 12.9

Occupational contact dermatitis of hands of a dialysis-technician who showed patch test positivity to formaldehyde

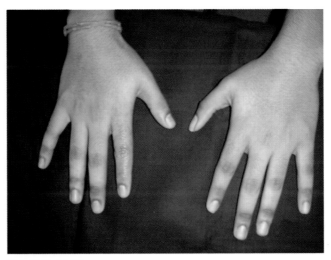

FIGURE 12.10

Occupational contact dermatitis of hands of an aquarium-cleaner who used detergents to clean the aquarium

13 Chemical Leukoderma

DEFINITION

Chemical leukoderma represents an acquired vitiligo-like hypomelanosis induced by repeated (multiple) exposure to specific chemical compounds.

[This chemical effect, independent of their sensitizing potential, is distinctly separate from post-inflammatory depigmentation and Koebner phenomenon in vitiligo]

Terminology

☑ Chemical leukoderma

☐ Contact leukoderma

☐ Occupational leukoderma

[Proposal: The term 'chemical leukoderma' is more acceptable as:

1. The term 'contact leukoderma' may signify as if the mechanism of contact leukoderma is similar to contact dermatitis, which is not true

2. This leukoderma can also originate from household or daily-usage product apart from occupational chemical exposure]

(Ghosh, 2005)

Chemical Leukoderma : How a Chemical Exposure in Localised Area can Lead to Generalised Vitiliginous Process ?

4-TBP + Melanocyte ⟶ Oxidative stress
⟶ Release of stress protein
(Heat shock protein)
[HSP 70]
(inadequate for protection)

Induces
TRAIL-expression

Activates
DC effector functions

Systemic autoimmunity ⟵ ─── DC return to draining lymph node

[4-TBP: Para-tertiary butyl phenol; TRAIL: TNF-related apoptosis-induced ligand; DC: Dendritic cell]

(Kroll TM et al 2005, Boissy, 2006)

Clinical Features

- Vitiligo-like macules
- May spread to remote site (without direct or indirect contact)
- Confetti macules
- Symmetrical or asymmetrical
- Surrounding hyperpigmentation (occasionally) (leukomelanoderma)
- Irritant/allergic contact dermatitis is not a prerequisite

Chemical Leukoderma and Vitiligo: Clinical Comparison

	Chem leuko	Vitiligo
Trichrome color	–	+
Leukotrichia	–	+
Koebner	–	+
Confetti macules	+	–

Chemical Leukoderma versus Koebner in Vitiligo

	Chem leuko	Koebner
Exposure	Multiple	Single
Configuration	Any type	Usually linear
Pre-existing vitiligo	Absent	Present

Chemical Leukoderma versus Post-inflammatory Leukoderma

	Chem leuko	Post-inflammatory
Primary rash	Nil	Present
Limitation	May spread beyond the contact area	Limited to original site
Confetti macules	+	–

Chemical Leukoderma : Clinical Diagnostic Criteria (Proposed)

- Acquired vitiligo-like hypomelanosis induced by repeated exposure to specific chemical compound
- Patterned vitiligo-like macule is conforming to site of exposure
- Confetti macules

(Any two among the above-three criteria should be present simultaneously to diagnose chemical leukoderma clinically)

(Ghosh S, 2005)

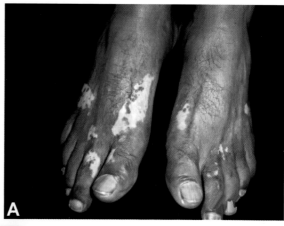

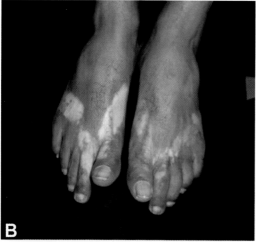

FIGURES 13.2A AND B

Chemical leukoderma on feet from using rubber chappal

Chemical Leukoderma: Contributory Chemicals	
Most potent phenol/catechol derivatives • Monobenzyl ether of hydroquinone (MBH) • Hydroquinone • p-tert-butylcatechol (PTBC) • p-tert-butylphenol (PTBP) • p-tert-amylphenol (PTAP) *Additional phenol/catechol derivatives* • Monomethyl ether of hydroquinone (MMH) • Monothyl ether of hydroquinone (MEH) • p-phenylphenol • p-octylphenol • p-cresol	*Sulfhydryls* • Cysteamine • Sulfanolic acid • Cystamina dihydrochloride *Miscellaneous* • Mercurials • Arsenic • Cinnamic aldehyde • Paraphenylene diamine (PPD) (Bajaj 1996) • Azo dye (Bajaj 2000) • Corticosteroids • Chloroquin • Soymilk and derived protein • Anmoniated mercury • Thiotepa

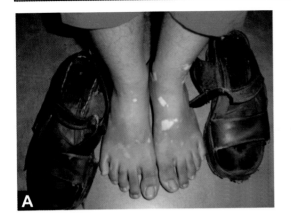

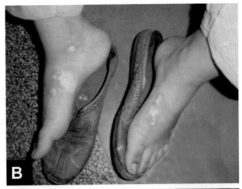

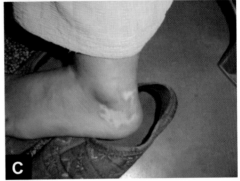

FIGURE 13.2A TO C

Chemical leukoderma of feet from PPD (paraphenylediamine) of shoe

Chemical Leukoderma: Common Sources	
Germicidal detergent	Rubber antioxidants
Varnish and lacquer resins	Motor oil additives
Synthetic oils	Deodorants
Duplicate paper	Formaldehyde resins
Soap antioxidants	Latex gloves
De-emulsifiers (oil-field)	Plasticizers
Insecticides	Printing inks
Disinfectants	Paints
Photographic chemicals	Adhesive

(Boissy and Manga, 2004)

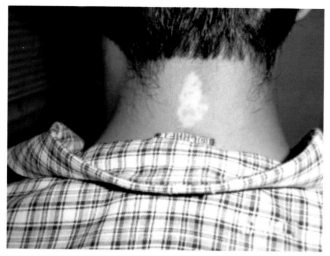

FIGURE 13.3
Chemical leukoderma of neck from the sticker of collar of the shirt

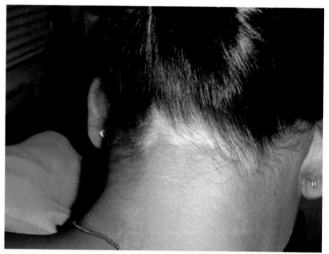

FIGURE 13.4
Chemical leukoderma from hair dye (PPD) on the neck

Chemical Leukoderma: Unique Sources
• Hair dye (PPD)
• Toothpaste (Cinnammic)
• Tattoo (PPD)
• Nickel
• Artificial nails (Methacrylate)
• Swim-goggles (Neoprene rubber/gloves)
• Rubber (Hawaian) Sandal (Mercaptobenzothiazol & Thiurams)
• Perfume
• Bindi (PTB) (Bajaj 1990)
• Wallet (Synthetic leather : MBH) [on breast of Indian ladies] (Bajaj 1991)
• Footwear
• Alta (feet decorative cosmetic) (Azo dye) (Bajaj 1998)
• Amulet string (Azo dye) (Banerjee 2004)

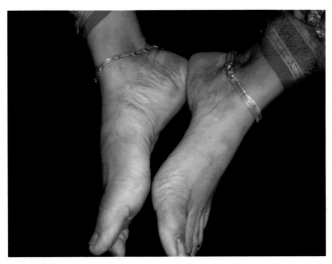

FIGURE 13.5

Chemical leukoderma on feet by using 'alta' (red coloring decorating paint used by Indian ladies)

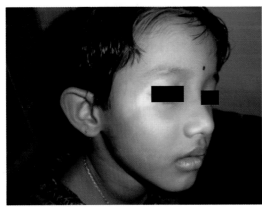

FIGURE 13.6

Chemical leukoderma of a child's face by using make-up containing ammoniated mercury

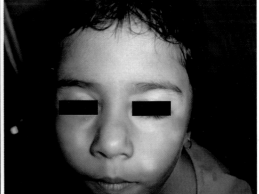

FIGURE 13.7

Chemical leukoderma of the face of a child by contact with the pillow of her grandmother using hair dye (PPD)

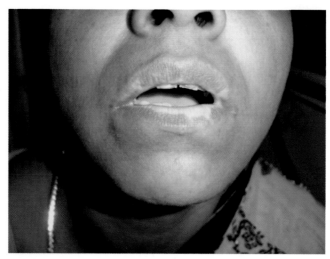

FIGURE 13.8

Chemical leukoderma on lip from lipstick containing azo dye

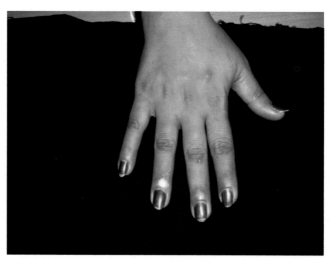

FIGURE 13.9

Chemical leukoderma of fingers by using nail polish from the lacquer resins

14 Photocontact Dermatitis

Photocontact dermatitis implies the dermatoses produced by some substances only in the presence of light.

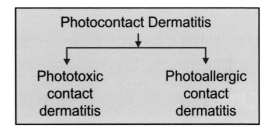

Photoallergic contact dermatitis (PACD) sometimes may superimpose on polymorphous light eruption (PLE).

Photoallergic and Phototoxic Contact Dermatitis : Comparison		
	Photoallergic	*Phototoxic*
Incidence	Low	High
Onset at first exposure	No	Yes
Onset after UV exposure	24-48 hr	Minutes to days
Dose dependence		
– Chemical	Not important	Important
– Radiation	Not important	Important
Clinical morphology	Eczematous	Erythema and edema, bullous, eczematous, urticarial, papular, pigmentation, lichenoid, pseudo-porphyric
Route of exposure		
– Topical	+++	++
– Systemic	+	+++
		(After Marks, Elsner, DeLeo, 2002)

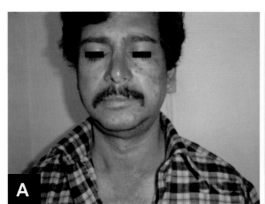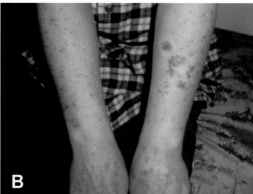

FIGURES 14.1A AND B

Phototoxic contact dermatitis of a person who works with different dye in a printing press

Phototoxic Contact Dermatitis: Contributory Important Agents	
Coal Tar Derivatives • Coal tar • Pitch • Creosote *Furocoumarins* • Psoralens • Fig • Orange • Carrot • Celery • Parsley • Parsnip • Bergamot • Meadow grass	*Dyes* • Eosin • Methylene blue • Toluidine blue • Acridine orange • Acriflavine • Rose Bengal • Neutral red • Disperse blue 35

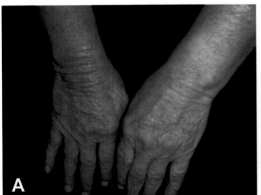 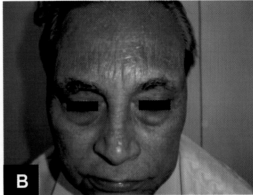

FIGURES 14.2A AND B

Photoallergic contact dermatitis of a person who used to apply soap containing antiseptic agent triclosan

Photoallergic Contact Dermatitis : Contributory Important Agents	
Sunscreen Agents • Para-amino benzoic acid (PABA) esters • Benzophenones (oxybenzone) • Cinnamates	*Antibacterial Agents* • Chlorhexidine • Triclosan • Dichlorophene
Fragrances • Musk ambrette • 6-Methylcoumarin • Sandalwood oil	*Therapeutic Agents* • Ketoprofen gel • Promethazine (topical) • Chlorpromazine hydrochloride (topical handling)

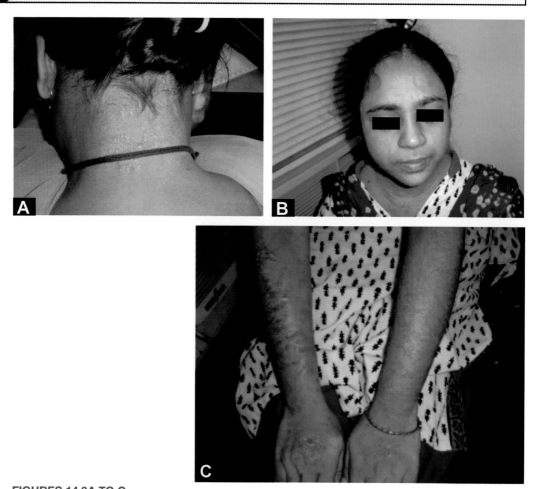

FIGURES 14.3A TO C

Photoallergic contact dermatitis of a lady on back of neck, face and forearms by using perfume containing musk ambrette

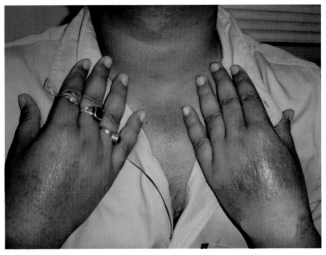

FIGURE 14.4

Photoallergic contact dermatitis of a compounder on dorsum of hands and V-area of neck from handling chlorpromazine while injecting into the patient

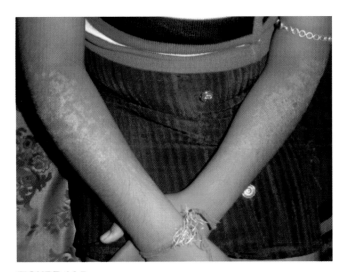

FIGURE 14.5

Photoallergic contact dermatitis in a lady on both forearms from using sunscreen containing oxybenzone

PHOTOPATCH TEST

Photopatch test is an useful diagnostic test to detect photoallergic contact dermatitis.

Photopatch Test: Method

Day 0 A portion of the lower back is marked and exposed to UVA lights at a dose of 5J/cm² (Photo-testing).

The test site, usually the upper back is selected, where the photoallergens, in two sets, are placed on both the sides. The common photoallergens with control are applied by Finn chambers.

Day 1 (After 24 hours) : The patch on the left side is removed and the patch test reading is taken. The right side (non-irradiated side) is then covered with an opaque dark covering. The left side is then exposed to UVA at a dose of 5J/cm² (irradiated side). The patch at the right side is then removed. Both the sides are marked accordingly with the marker pen.

Day 2 (After 72 hours) : Reading on the both sides are noted. Offending allergens causing photocontact dermatitis or allergic contact dermatitis are identified. Post-photopatch test counselling is done and then instruction is given to avoid individual allergen accordingly.

Photopatch Test: Indication

Eczematous eruption predominantly affecting light-exposed sites and in whom a history of worsening occurs following light exposure.

Some authors recommend that all photosensitive patients should be photopatch tested.

(Marks, Elsner, DeLeo 2002)

Photopatch Test : Contraindication

- Systemic lupus erythematosus (SLE)

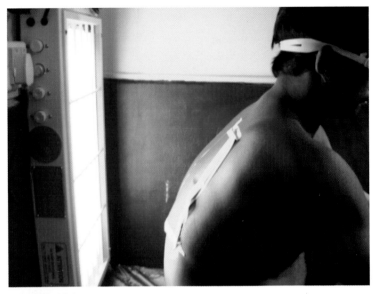

FIGURE 14.6

Photopatch test being done in a patient

Photopatch Test: Series of Common Photoallergens

A. Sunscreen
1. Para-amino benzoic acid (PABA)
2. Padimate O and A
3. Parsol MCX
4. Oxybenzone
5. Parsol 1789
6. Benzophenone
B. Fragrance ingredients
1. Musk ambrette
2. 6-Methyl coumarin
3. Sandalwood oil
C. Antibacterial agent
1. Buclosamide
2. Hexachlorophene
3. Halogenated salicylanides

D. Miscellaneous compounds
1. Patients' own products
2. Benzocaine
3. Chlorhexidine
4. Chlorpromazine
5. Diphenhydramine
6. Hydrocortisone
7. Promethazine
8. Thiourea
9. Paraphenylenediamine

15 Contact Dermatitis: Differential Diagnosis

Contact dermatitis may simulate many dermatoses very closely. Detailed history, clinical findings, certain pathological tests and patch test can differentiate between these diseases.

Contact Dermatitis: Differential Diagnosis

- Atopic dermatitis
- Seborrheic dermatitis
- Psoriasis
- Tinea infection
- Polymorphous light eruption (PLE)

ATOPIC DERMATITIS

Salient Features

- Usually onset at childhood
- Family history of atopy (allergic rhinitis, bronchial asthma, allergic conjunctivitis)
- Personal history of atopy
- High IgE level (usually)
- Infants : Extensor aspect of the limbs affected
- Older children/adults : flexural aspect more affected
- Fulfil major and minor criteria of atopic dermatitis

Atopic Dermatitis (AD) and Systemic Reaction of Contact Dermatitis (SRCD)		
	AD	SRCD
Onset	Childhood	Adulthood
Family history	Usually +ve	–ve
IgE	Usually high	Normal
Patch test to offending allergens	–ve	+ve

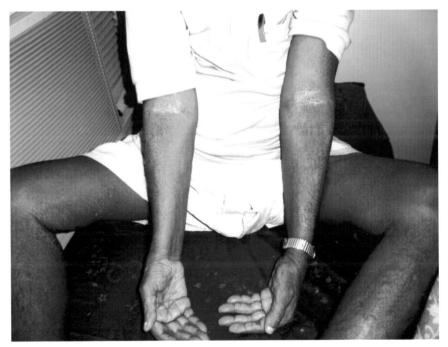

FIGURE 15.1

Atopic dermatitis of an adult involving flexors of the limbs

SEBORRHEIC DERMATITIS

Salient Features

- Greasy scales or erythematous scaly dermatitis on scalp, face (eyebrows, beard area, nasolabial furrows), front and back of chest, axillae, groin and flexors
- First six to nine months of age and then after puberty age group
- Occasionally familial.

Seborrheic Dermatitis and Airborne Contact Dermatitis: Comparison		
	Seborrheic Dermatitis	*Airborne Contact Dermatitis*
Age	Infancy, puberty, adult	Not in infancy
History	No h/o aero-allergens	H/o aero-allergens
Patch test	–ve	+ve

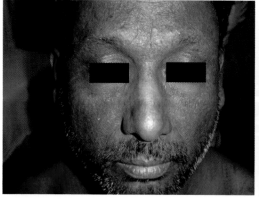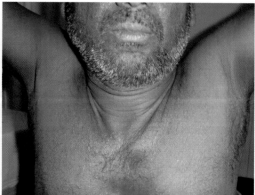

FIGURE 15.2

Seborrheic dermatitis of a patient involving face and axillae

PSORIASIS

Salient Features

- Silver dry scales on scalp, extensor aspect of limbs, palmoplantar area or lower back
- Well-defined border
- Guttate psoriasis are dew-drop like generalized eruption with minimal scales
- Auspitz sign +ve
- Nail pitting and other nail changes
- Occasionally arthropathy
- Patch test negative.

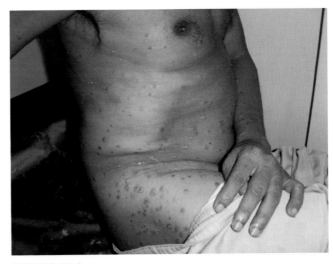

FIGURE 15.3

Guttate psoriasis in a man

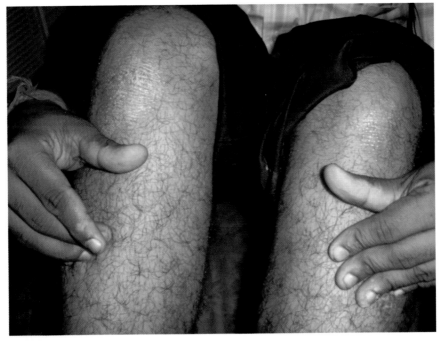

FIGURE 15.4

Psoriasis involving fingers and extensor aspect of knee

TINEA INFECTION

Salient Features

- Inflammatory active border and central clearing
- Characteristic nail changes occasionally
- Usually unilateral
- Skin scraping or nail clipping shows positive fungal smear (by KOH)
- Patch test negative.

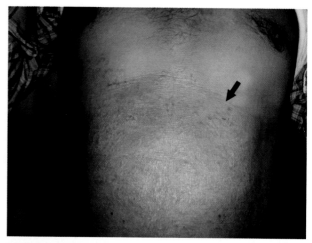

FIGURE 15.5
Tinea corporis of abdomen with active border

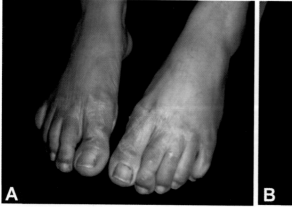
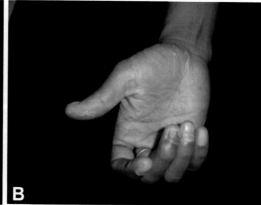

FIGURES 15.6A AND B
Tinea pedis and tinea manum with onychomycosis of same person showing active border

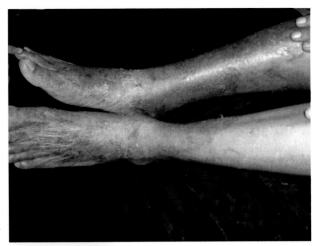

FIGURE 15.7

Tinea of feet with active border

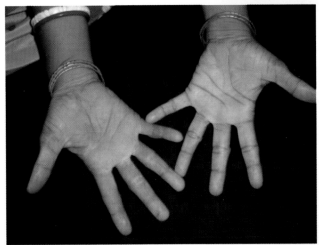

FIGURE 15.8

Tinea of hands with active border involving one hand mostly interdigital areas

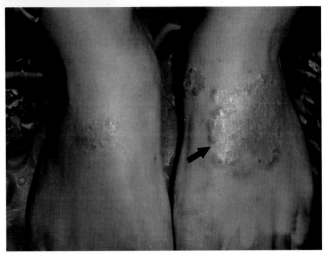

FIGURE 15.9

Tinea on dorsum of feet showing active border and central clearing

POLYMORPHOUS LIGHT ERUPTION

Salient Features

- Eczematous eruption on exposed skin, i.e. dorsum of hand and feet, forehead, V-area of neck
- No history of contact with photo-allergens
- Photopatch test negative.

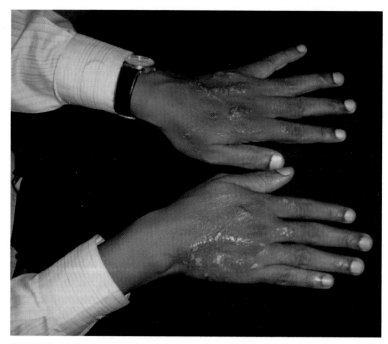

FIGURE 15.10

Polymorphous light eruption on dorsum of hands, photopatch test being negative

Complications of Contact Dermatitis

Contact dermatitis, though apparently innocuous disease, may occasionally give rise to complications, some of which are major.

Contact Dermatitis: Complications
• Secondary infection
• Lymphangitis
– Acute
– Recurrent
• Cellulitis
• Post-inflammatory hyperpigmentation
• Post-inflammatory hypopigmentation

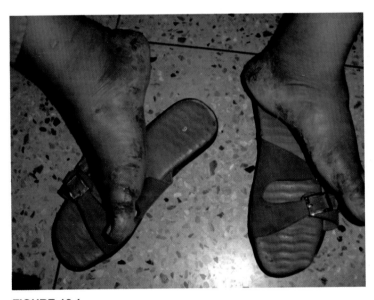

FIGURE 16.1
Allergic contact dermatitis on feet from footwear got secondarily infected with bacteria

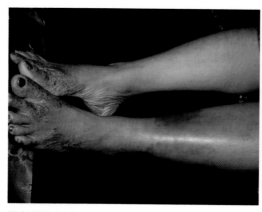

FIGURE 16.2

Acute lymphangitis from contact dermatitis of foot caused by footwear

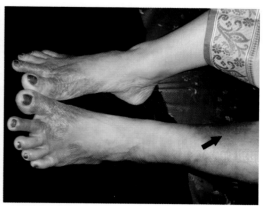

FIGURE 16.3

Acute lymphangitis, occurring recurrently, contact dermatitis from footwear being the source

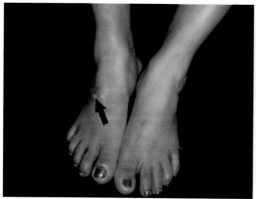

FIGURE 16.4

Contact dermatitis from footwear causing post-inflammatory depigmentation

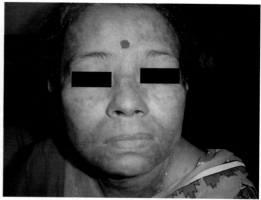

FIGURE 16.5

Contact dermatitis from cosmetic cream causing secondary post-inflammatory hyperpigmentation

Management of Contact Dermatitis

A) Treatment

1) Acute lesions   : Topical steroid lotion

    Subacute lesions : Topical steroid cream or pimecrolimus cream

    Chronic lesions : Topical steroid ointment or tacrolimus ointment.

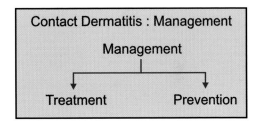

Contact Dermatitis : Management

(Belsito DV, Fitzpatrick's Dermatology in General Medicine, 2003)

[Long continued potent, regular or intermittent topical steroid can cause atrophy of skin and thus can create more defect in its barrier function (Anderson KE, 2005). This can lead to more penetration of irritants or allergens into the epidemis making the contact dermatitis more persistent. Hence after providing the primary relief with potent topical steroid the treatment is to be continued with either low potent topical steroid or pimecrolimus or tacrolimus]

2) Oral antibiotics, when signs of secondary infection or associated lymphangitis or cellulitis seen.

3) Oral anti-histamines to alleviate itching, irritation, if associated.

4) Short courses of oral corticosteroids in case of severe contact dermatitis.

5) In case of refractory contact dermatitis, following remedies can be attempted:
   - UVB-NB
   - PUVA
   - Azathioprine [100-150 mg/d × 6 month in airborne parthenium dermatitis] (Sharma, 1998)
   - Cyclosporin [5 mg/kg/d] (Higgins, 1991).

B) Prevention

1) Identification of irritants and allergens by history or patch test and avoidance or use of substitute substances, where possible.

2) Identification of cross-reacting allergens, if any and avoidance or use of substitute substances, where possible.

3) Emollients to be used liberally to prevent dryness of skin. This will help restoration of barrier function of the skin. Emollients should be paraben-free, lanolin-free and fragrance-free (Sen M, Mukhopadhaya S, Ghosh S, 2006).

4) Use of soap substitute which helps to prevent further damage of epidermal barrier function (Nixon RL, 2002).

5) Liberal use of barrier creams will help in prevention of contact of offending substances to some extent.

6) Gloves should be used by the sufferer, where possible. In case of rubber allergy one can use cotton or polythene gloves beneath the rubber gloves.

Contact Dermatitis : Prevention

- Identification and avoidance of irritants/allergens
- Identification and avoidance of cross-reacting allergens, if any
- Emollient
- Soap substitutes
- Barrier cream
- Gloves

Allergens : Sources, Cross-reaction, Skin Lesions and Substitute				
Allergen	*Sources*	*Cross-reaction*	*Skin lesion*	*Substitute/ alternatives*
1. Potassium dichromate	Cement, Tanned leather, Textile dyes, Wood preservative, Alloy in metal, Safety match, Photography, Electroplating. Anticorrosive, Engraving and lithography, Ceramics, Automobile industries, TV manufacturing, Photocopy paper, Tattoos, Mascara, Eye shadows, Welding, Milk testing, Floor waxes, Shoe polishes, Painting glue, Pigments, Detergents		Allergic contact dermatitis (ACD) Airborne contact dermatitis	Freshly prepared ferrous sulfate may be added to convert potassium dichromate to potassium bichromate which penetrates less into the skin Low hexavalent chromate cement Vegetable tanned leather Chrom-free leather
2. Neomycin sulfate	Topical antibiotics used in skin, eye, ear treatment; veterinary use	Streptomycin Gentamycin Framycetin Dihydrostrepto-mycin Kanamycin Spectinomycin Tobramycin Bacitracin	ACD	
3. Cobalt chloride-hexahy-drate	Paints for glass and porcelain, Jewellery, Zippers, Button, Tools, Utensils, Instrument, Hair dyes, Cosmetics, Dental appliances		ACD, Airborne contact dermatitis, Erythema multiforme	
4. Benzocaine	Local and topical anesthetic agents, Hemorrhoidal cream, Suppository, Oral and gingival products, Sore throat sprays/lozenges, Astringent, Appetite suppressants	Paragroup of compound, Ethylenediamine, Procainamide Hypochlorothiaz-ide, PABA & ester, Azo/ aniline dyes, PPD, Sulfonamides, Sulfonylureas, Aminosalicylic acid, Parabens		

Contd...

Contd...

Allergen	Sources	Cross-reaction	Skin lesion	Substitute/ alternatives
5. 4-pheny-lene diamine (PPD)	Permanent hair dye, Fur dyes, Photographic developer, Lithography, Photocopying, Oils, Greases, Gasoline, Antioxidant, Accelerator in the rubber and plastic items, Blood reagents	PABA, Para compounds	ACD, Airborne contact dermatitis, Erythema multiforme	
6. Parabens	Preservative in food, Cosmetics, Medicaments, Oils, Fats, Glues, Shoe polish	Other parabens, Hydroquinone, Monobenzyl ether of hydroquinone, Paragroup of compounds		
7. Nickel sulfate hexahydrate	Alloys, Electroplated metal, Earring, Watches, Button, Zipper, Rings, Utensils, Tools, Instrument, Batteries, Machinery parts, Metal cutting fluid, Nickel plates, Coins, Pigments, Dentures, Orthopedic plates, Keys, Scissors, Razors, Spectacle frame, Kitchen utensils		ACD, Airborne CD	High quality stainless steel, Sterling silver, Platinum or Titanium or other metal (watch, watch band, spectacle frame), Several layers of clean nail polish on daily-using nickel objects (like keys, scissors) can be applied repeatedly to prevent release of nickel
8. Colophony	Varnishes, Printing inks, Paper, Glues, Tackifiers, Adhesive, Surface coating, Polish, Waxes, Cosmetics (mascara, rouge, eye shadow), Topical medicament, Violin bow resin, Athletes grip-aid	Balsam of Peru, Wood tars, Dihydro abietyl alcohol	ACD, Airborne contact dermatitis	
9. Gentamicin sulfate	Topical & systemic antibiotics, Eye/ear drops	Neomycin sulfate	ACD	

Contd...

Contd...

Allergen	Sources	Cross-Reaction	Skin Lesion	Substitute/ alternatives
10. Mercepto-Mix	Accelerator in natural and some synthetic rubber, Retarders for chloropene rubber		ACD	
11. Epoxy resin	Adhesives, Surface coating, Electrical insulation, Plasticizers, Polymer stabilizer, Laminates, Surface coating, Paints and inks, Product finishes, PVC products, Vinyl gloves, Sculptures		ACD, Airborne contact dermatitis, Erythema multiforme	
12. Fragrance Mix	Soap, Perfume, Toothpaste, Colognes, After shave lotion, Scents, Food items like sweets, ice cream, chewing gums, soft drinks, Room freshners, Insect Repellents			Fragrance-free cosmetics and medicaments
13. Mercep-tobenzoth-iazole	Accelerator, retarder and peptizer of natural and other rubber products, Shoes, Gloves, Undergarments, Clothing, Condom, Diaphragm, Medical devices, Toys, Tyres, Fungicide, Corrosive inhibitor, Insoluble cutting oils, Detergent, Tick and flea powder, Spray		ACD	
14. Nitrofura-zone	Topical medicaments in human and veterinary medicines, Animal feeds		ACD, Airborne contact dermatitis	
15. 4-chloro-3-cresol (chlorocresol)	Fungicidal cream, Topical antiseptic, Pharmaceutical product, Protein shampoo, Baby cosmetics, Cooling fluids, Adhesives and glues, Inks, Paints, Varnishes, Packing materials, Tanning agents	4-chloro-3 xylenenol (Dettol)	ACD	

Contd...

Contd...

Allergen	Sources	Cross-reaction	Skin lesion	Substitute/ alternatives
16. Wool alcohol (Lanolin)	Cosmetics, Pharmaceuticals, Moisturizers, Emollient, Emulsifying preparation, Topical drugs, Furniture polish, Leather, Paper, Metal corrosive prevention, Inks, Textiles, Furs, Cutting oil, Waxes, Oil emulsions			
17. Balsam of Peru	Flavor in Tobacco, Drinks, Pastries, Cakes, Wine, Liqueur, Spices, Fixative and fragrances in perfumery, Topical medicament, Dentistry	Balsam of tolu, Cinnamate, Benzoates, Styrax, Benzoin, Tiger balm, Coniferyl alcohol, Coumarin, Eugenol, Isoeugenol Propolis, Propanidid, Diethylstibe- sterol		
18. Thiuram Mix	Accelerator, activator of natural rubber and other synthetic rubber, Fungicidal, Disinfectants for seeds, Bacteriostatic in soap, Animal repellents, Disulfiram			
19. Chinoform	Antiinfective and antiamebic agents in topical or oral medicine, Graphic developers, Lithography, Photocopying, Oils, Greases, Gasoline, Antioxidant in rubber and plastic industry	Parabens, PABA, Para compounds	ACD, Airborne CD, Erythema multiforme	

Contd...

Contd...

Allergen	Sources	Cross-reaction	Skin lesion	Substitute/ alternatives
20. Black Rubber Mix	Antioxidants and antiozonants in rubber, Tyres, Tubes, Pipe gas flays, Black rubber shoes, Gloves, Sole, Earphones, Walking stick handles, Squash balls, Face masks, Eyelash curler, Wood surfers.		ACD	
21. P-tert-butyl phenol formal-dehyde resin	Resin used in adhesives of shoes, bindies, watch strap, Self glues, Plywood, Insulation, Automobiles, Motor oils, Inks, Paper Film developers, Disinfectants, Deodorants		ACD, May cause depig-mentation	
22. Formalde-hyde	Production of urea, Astringents, Disinfectants, Preservatives in cosmetics, Antiperspirants, Chipboard production, Dry Cleaning materials, Crease-free textiles, Adhesives, Footwear polishes, Medicine, Embalming solution		ACD, Air borne CD, Erythema multiforme	
23. Poly-ethylene glycol 400	Cosmetics (shampoo, hair dressing), Topical emollient, Detergents, Toothpaste, Insect repellents		ACD	

[After Indian Standard Battery of Allergens by Contact and Occupational Dermatoses Forum of India (CODFI, 2005)]

Cross-reaction between Chemicals and Foods (may cause Systemic Reactivation of Contact Dermatitis or SRCD)

Chemicals	Foods
Latex	Banana, tomato, potato, avocado, Kiwi
Nickel	Steel (low quality) plate, glass used for food and drinks, tinned food, beans, corn, spinach, peas, mushroom, peanuts
Balsam of Peru	Citrus fruits, spices, condiments, pickles, wine, beer, gin, chocolate, cola drinks, tomato

Nickel Release Spot Test (Fisher Test)

- A screening test for nickel release from any suspected nickel objects
- Method: After rubbing the surface with cotton wool-tipped stick soaked with two drops of DMG (dimethylgly-oxime), red or pink color develops.

Management: Occupational Dermatitis

- Treatment
  - As described in contact dermatitis
- Prevention
  - Pre-employment screen for identification of high risk population
  - Hazardous material identification
  - Factory visit by derma-allergologists
- Public health measures
  - Employer : Technical means, Quality control, House keeping,
                Warning, Education, Monitoring
  - Worker : Personal protection, Hygiene, Education, Awareness
  - Government : Quality, Industry regulation, Control, Education and awareness
  - Medical : Recognition, Early therapy, Education

Management: Photocontact Dermatitis

A. Avoidance of photoallergens
B. Physical   : Clothing,
                   Hat, Umbrella,
                   Full sleeves
C. Sunscreen : Chemical sunscreen,
                   Sunblocker/physical sunscreen,
                   Combination
D. Systemic   : Beta-carotene,
                   Antimalarial drug, e.g. Chloroquine/Hydroxychloroquine,
                   PUVA,
                   UVB-NB

Management: Chemical Leukoderma

- Counselling to detect the offending agents
- Strict and permanent removal of cause
- PUVA (topical or systemic)
- UVB-NB
- Prognosis
  - Early cases: good (if cause withdrawn totally)
  - After repigmentation, recurrence rare.

Bibliography

1. Adams RM, Maibach HI. A five year study of cosmetic reaction. J Am Acad Dermatol 1985;13:1062-9.
2. Anderson KE. The diagonsis and treatment of occupational hand eczema. Abstract, 33rd National Conference of IADVL and 4th South Asian Regional Conference of Dermatology and Leprology, New Delhi 2005;3-6:39.
3. Bajaj AK, Gupta SC, Chatterjee AK, Singh KG. Shoe dermatitis in India. Contact Dermatitis 1988;19:371-5.
4. Bajaj AK, Sareswat A. Systemc contact dermatitis. Ind J Dermatol Venereol Leprol 2006;72:99-102.
5. Bajaj AK. Contact dermatitis. In : IADVL Textbook of Dermatology Vol 1, 2nd ed, Ed Valia RG. Mumbai:Bhalani 2001;453-97.
6. Bajaj AK. Patch Testing:An Overview. In : Recent Advances in Dermatology. Ed S Ghosh. New Delhi:Jaypee 2004;136-46.
7. Bajaj AK, Gupta SC, Chatterjee AK. Contact depigmentation from free paratertiary butyl phenol in bindi adhesive. Contact Dermatitis 1990; 22:99-102.
8. Bajaj AK, Gupta SC, Chatterjee AK. Depigmentation of the breast. Contact Dermatitis 1991; 24:58.
9. Bajaj AK, Gupta SC, Chatterjee AK, et al. Hair dye depigmentation. Contact Dermatitis 1996; 35:56-7.
10. Bajaj AK, Pandey RK, Misra K, et al. Contact depigmentation caused by an azo dye in alta. Contact Dermatitis 1998; 38:189-93.
11. Bajaj AK, Mishra A, Misra K, et al. The azo dye solvent yellow 3 produces depigmentation. Contact Dermatitis 2000;42:237-8.
12. Banerjee K, Banerjee R, Mondal B. Amulet string contact leukoderma and its differentiation from vitiligo. J Dermatal Venereol Leprol 2004;70180-1.
13. Boissy RE, Monga P. On the etiology of contact/occupational vitiligo. Pigment Cell Research 2004;17(3):208-14.
14. Belsito DV. Allergic Contact Dermatitis. In: Fitzpatrick's Dermatology in General Medicine. Ed. Freedberg IM, et al. McGrraw Hill: New York, 2003;1164-77.
15. British Photodermatology group : Workshop report on photopatch testing methods and indication. Brit J Dermatology 1997;136:371-6.
16. Chowdhuri S, Ghosh S. Epidemio-allergological study in 155 cases of footwear dermatitis. Indian J Dermatol venereol leprol 2007;319-22.
17. Fisher AA. Contact Dermatitis (3rd edn), Lea & Febiger: Philadelphia 1986.
18. Ghosh S, Sarma N, Mukhopadhaya S. Airborne contact dermatitis: Clinico-allergological study in sixtyfour cases. Abstracts, The Asia-pacific Environmental & Occupational Dermatology Symposium. Philippines; Manila 2005; 45.

19. Ghosh S. Clinico-etiological study of chemical leukoderma. Abstact, 7th Asian Congress of Dermatology, Kuala Lumpur 2005;223.
20. Goh CL, Wong WK, Ng SK. Comparison between 1-day and 2-day occlusion times in patch testing. Contact dermatitis 1994,31:48-9.
21. Gordon LA. Composite dermatitis. Australasian J of Dermatology 1999;40(3):123-30.
22. Hawelia D. Lichenoid contact dermatitis, Bulletin of IAISD, 2006;1:3.
23. Higgins EM, McLelland J, Friedman PS, et al. Oral cyclosporin inhibits the expression of contact hypersensitivity in man. J Dermatol Sci. 1991;2:79-83.
24. Handa F, Handa S, Handa R. Environment factors and the skin. In. IADVL Text Book and Atlas of Dermatology. Vol 1. Ed. R G Valia, Bhalani, Mumbai 2001;81-91.
25. Ket NS, Leok GC. The Principles and Practice of Contact and Occupational Dermatology in the Asia-Pacific Region, World Scientific, New Jersey, 2001.
26. Kim E, Maibach H. Contact urticaria. In:Urticaria and Angioedema. Ed Greaves MW, Keplan AP, New York:Marcel 2004;149-69.
27. Kroll TM, Bommiasamy H, Boissy RE et al. 4-tertary butyl phenol exposures sensitizes human melonocytes to dendritic cell-mediated killing : Relevance to vitiligo. J of Invest Dermatology 2005;124(4):798-806.
28. Lachapelle JM, Maibach HI. Patch Testing Prick Testing : A Practical Guide. Springer:Berlin, 2003.
29. Manuskiatti W, Maibach HI. 1 versus 2 and 3-day diagnostics patch testing. Contact Dermatitis 1996;35:97-200.
30. Marks JG, Elsner P, De Leo V. Contact & Occupational Dermatology, 3rd Ed, Mosby:London 2002.
31. Nandakishore TH, Pasricha JS. Pattern of cross sensitity between four compositae plants parthenium hysterophorus, Xanthium strumarium, Helianthus annuusm and Chrysanthemum coronarium in Indian patients. Contact Dermatitis 1994;30:162-7.
32. Nixon RL. Allergic contact dermatitis and photoallergy. In Lebwohl M (Ed). Mosby: London. Treatment of Skin Disease 2002;22-25.
33. Pasricha JS, Verma KK. Special problems and perspective from India. Quoted in : No. 25.
34. Rietschel R. (1990) in Irritant contact dermatitis Eds Jackson EM, Goldman R Quoted in No 30.
35. Saha M, Srinivas CR. Footwear dermatitis possibly due to paraphylenediamine in socks. Dermatologica 1985;170:260-2.
36. Sarma N, Ghosh S. Clinico-epidemiological profile of paraphenylendiamine sensitivity. Abstract, 34th National Conference of IADVL, 1-5 Feb 2006, 171.
37. Sarma N. Clinical features and special types of urticaria. In : Urticaria Update. Ed. S. Ghosh, Kolkata:IAISD, 2005;18-47.
38. Sharma VK, Chakrabarti A, Mahajan V, Azathioprine in the treatment of parthenium dermatitis. Int J Dermatol 1998;37:299-302.
39. Sen M, Mukhopadhyaya S, Ghosh S. Paraben, Lanolin, Fragrance allergy : A Clinico-Epidemiological Study. Abstract, 34th National Conference of IADVL, Hyderabad 1-5 Feb 2006; 172.
40. Wahlberg JE, Elsner P, Kanerva L, Maibach HI. Management of Positive Patch Test Reaction. Springer:Berlin 2003.
41. Wilkinson DS, Fregret S, Magnusson B, et al. Terminology of contact dermatitis. Acta Dermato-Venereologica 1970;50:287.

Index